TALES FROM ANOTHER

Mother Runner

Other Books by
Dimity McDowell and Sarah Bowen Shea

Run Like a Mother: How to Get Moving—
and Not Lose Your Family, Job, or Sanity

Train Like a Mother: How to Get Across Any Finish Line—
and Not Lose Your Family, Job, or Sanity

TALES FROM ANOTHER
Mother Runner

Triumphs, Trials, Tips, and Tricks from the Road

A Collection from Badass Mother Runners

Edited by Dimity McDowell and Sarah Bowen Shea

Andrews McMeel Publishing®

Kansas City · Sydney · London

Pamela--
You are awesome
for spreading the
AMR love.
xo _SBS

Pamela—
Many more
happy miles!
xo—
Dimity

To certified—and aspiring—

BAMRs everywhere

CONTENTS

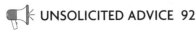

TALES FROM ANOTHER

Mother Runner

INTRODUCTION

I, Dimity, am in mile 21 of the Nike Women's Marathon with my sister Sarah by my side. By all accounts, we're probably looking pretty capable for just having run for more than three hours. I'm a spritely thirty-four, Sarah is five years younger, and we're charging as fast as mid-pack marathon runners do toward the finish line. (Read: Walk breaks, previously reserved for aid stations, now happen randomly and often.) I might even look cute. My long legs are sleek from miles of marathon training, I got an expensive haircut less than a week ago, and I'm wearing a black running dress, which is as *Project Runway* as running gear gets. Okay, wavy, white sweat lines decorate the dress pits, and a Team in Training coach—not my coach, mind you—on the sidelines just told me to shake out my arms, so I'm clearly not the picture of Perfect Running Form, but all things considered? Capable and cute.

On the inside though, I've fallen apart. I don't think I'll ever see the finish line, and quite frankly, I have no interest in getting there. "This sucks. This sucks. This sucks," is on repeat in my head, not quite the *you-can-do-it* mantra I need. I'm not listening to music, so I can't power up Gwen Stefani and her B-A-N-A-N-A-S to get me through. I'm D-O-N-E. The finisher's silver Tiffany necklace waiting for me at the end is about as enticing as a plastic spider ring given out on Halloween in lieu of candy. Don't. Want. It.

All I want? To not have to run another step. Ever again. Sarah is no help. In her own world of hurt, she gets mad at me when I set a modest goal (run thirty feet to that cone, then we can walk) and bail on it twenty feet into the challenge. "You can't do that, Ditty!" she complains. "Not fair." Her words sting as much as my left hip, which has flared up like a firecracker.

Although mile 21 of any marathon isn't a particularly pleasant place to be, our situation is worse because we went out too fast. Much too fast. Our first miles were in the low eights, a very ambitious pace for most, and ridiculously so for me; my longest training run was 16 miles because of a mid-training stress fracture in my left heel. Despite knowing better as we cruised through the first miles, I kept thinking, "This is awesome! We're flying *and* banking time." You can't bank time in a running race any more than you can open a savings account that pays 25 percent interest.

But rational thought has no place at a marathon party when I'm wearing a cute dress and a sassy haircut; when my sister, who makes me laugh like nobody else, is by my side; and when the crisp, fresh air of hip San Francisco makes me believe anything, including twenty-six consecutive eightish-minute splits, is possible.

Until I hit mile 21, and all I can think is, "WTF? Why am I doing this?"

As I hobble along, I can't recall the reasons I'm out here. All I can concentrate on is how much my leg hurts and how stupidly far 26.2 miles is to go. Rewind, though, and I was running 26.2 because I needed to get as far away as I could from postpartum depression, which hung over me after my second kid was born like the fog that almost always clouds San Francisco Bay. I was running 26.2 because if I didn't have a goal, a reason to throw back my covers in the morning and get my endorphins flowing, I wasn't confident I'd find my way back to some happier version of myself, the self that wanted to engage with my husband, my friends, the world. I was running 26.2 because it meant a weekend with my sister, and my friends Sarah and Katherine, during which I'd laugh, achieve, celebrate, shop, and, I hoped, feel joy—and kind of human again.

I wanted and needed it all so badly that after the podiatrist diagnosed the fracture and I stopped at Wendy's for a feel-better Frosty (not surprisingly, it didn't make me feel better), I immediately got on the phone with my coach to come up with a plan B. The fracture was bad enough that it should've ended my marathon goal, but that simply wasn't an option. I didn't want to watch others race. I needed to go the distance myself.

After trailing Dimity's easy-to-spot, 6' 4", dress-wearing figure since mile 9, I, Sarah (her friend, not her sister), am less than a quarter-mile behind her, and I am having my own marathon-inspired pity party. Thanks to sun and heat more often associated with L.A. than San Francisco, my white tech tee is heavy with sweat. I'm trendy, too, with my running skirt, but my thighs are having a shouting match, arguing over which one is in more pain from chub-rub. A hydration pack around my waist has chafed a raw spot on my lower back that probably is only the size of a quarter but feels like a pancake of pain. My marathon coach, Paula, a few feet ahead of me, is as perky and wiry as a Chihuahua; every few steps, she yips an upbeat, "Stay strong, Sarah; you've got this. You're doing great, girlfriend!"

Which is a whopper of a lie, but I'll get to that in a minute.

I'd stepped onto my Portland-to-San Francisco flight with my head and heart bulging with intentions to break the four-hour mark in the marathon. Paula had trained me for this, my fourth marathon, with the bold goal of having a finish time that started with a three. It was a goal I'd lusted for since I ran my first 26.2 as a divorced woman with no kids who was newly in love with Jack, a former college classmate. I'm not sure where I even got the idea of a sub-four-hour marathon; I didn't become athletic until college. Back in the 1990s, I considered myself a rower who sometimes ran, not a runner. I didn't even have many friends who had run a 26.2-mile race: My work-pal Dimity had run the 2007 New York City Marathon, and I had no clue what her finish time was. (*I, Dimity, do. It was 4:23. Or 4:32. One of those.*)

To the outside world, I had a sports swagger worthy of a first-round draft pick, often working into conversation boasts of top-five finishes at the highly competitive Head of the Charles rowing regatta. Yet 99 percent of it was bravado. Under a tough veneer of egotism was a marshmallow-soft center of self-doubt. To this day, every workout I do, every mile I run, fills chips in the veneer that threaten to reveal my true identity: a reader, not a rower or runner. I come from a long line of "people of the word," as my gentle Southern father likes to remind us. Since I feel exercise isn't wired into my DNA, I have to supplement it—and sometimes overdose on it—to compensate for a lack of genetic predisposition.

A sub-four marathon would validate my swagger, authenticate my bravado, and quiet my concerns about being a poser. It would make me a well-read runner, not a reader who runs. A swift marathon would show even though I'd crossed the line into my forties, I could be stronger, speedier, and maybe even a smidge sassier than I'd been pre-kids. It would prove even though I drove a minivan and carried a diaper bag, I still had a little *somethin' somethin'*.

For this marathon, I'd put my lofty time goal out into the blogosphere for all to see; Dimity and I wrote about our training on the *Runner's World* website as the Marathon Moms. (I married Jack and had three kids: one daughter, then five years old, and boy/girl twins, age two.) As I slog through each sunny mile, I can feel the goal slip from my sweaty grasp. The hills in the first half are my undoing, slowing me down and draining my energy. In Golden Gate Park, when my friend Christy bikes alongside me toward the halfway point, where my GPS reads 2:02, I admit out loud to her—and, really, to myself—the race isn't going as I'd hoped. My shoulders slump; my gut roils. I'd known this truth since (hilly) mile 5 or 6, but uttering the words feels dispiriting and disheartening.

As we circle Lake Merced, which somehow seems uphill all 5 miles around, I come to grips with the truth that's been staring me in the face since the park: I'm not going to finish anywhere close to four hours. Disappointment and dejection make each step feel even heavier than they already do. I'm angry at myself, at Paula, at Dimity for suggesting we run the race. Heck, I'm pissed at anyone who passes me because she has more juice left in her limbs than I do.

Near mile 22, Melissa Etheridge starts belting "I Run for Life" on my iPod. The breast-cancer survival anthem immediately reminds me of my brother's wife, who passed from the disease two years prior. I nearly stumble as I stifle a choking garble that wants to escape my throat. My tears mingle with sweat on my flushed cheeks, and I keep running.

Black dress on the outside and a sub-four goal: superficial stories that belie the real situations. Two variations on the make-it-stop theme on the inside: more honesty, more resonance. But the backstories? The most interesting—and most important—stories. The ones that make finish-line victories taste more delicious, invoke streams of tears, elicit smiles sweet as a peach.

A 1:59:58 half-marathon is damned impressive, especially when you hear the runner had massive GI issues starting at mile 4. But when you know the woman, despite losing her father three months earlier, was up at 4:30 a.m. for fourteen weeks through the Polar Vortex because she had to be showered and present for her special-needs child by 6:30 a.m.? Suddenly, you think she should've *won* the race.

Friend Sarah, bolstered by memories of her sister-in-law, passes my sister and me around mile 20. And I, Dimity, tough out those 5 miles. Because, well, what else was I really going to do? Stop and park myself on the curb? If it were Denver, my hometown, I might have, but it would've taken me at least five hours to find our hotel solo, so I keep marching toward the finish line. And I'm beyond thankful I did. Even with friend Sarah's 4:11 finish (a rockin' time, if you ask me), our account of running the Nike Women's Marathon solidified a mother-runner community that, during the next five years, becomes a staple for tens of thousands of women.

As we told tales of our miles and milestones in *Run Like a Mother* (2010) and dished out training and racing advice in *Train Like a Mother* (2012), we shared our backstories and carried a consistent tone that blended honesty, humor, inspiration, and support. The perspective in the chatty books spilled on to Facebook and our website, prompting a good friend to dub us the "Dear Abby for Mother Runners." And the chatter became our voices, as we started Another Mother Runner weekly podcasts. We coined a name for ourselves (Badass Mother Runners), complete with an acronym (BAMR) that isn't worthy of Merriam-Webster yet, but makes the hashtag rounds on Twitter, along with #motherrunner. What's more, the self-identifying shirts and tanks make appearances at races nationwide and are available at motherrunnerstore.com. (Maybe our next stop is QVC?)

Multitudes of other women around the country were doing exactly what we were doing: putting in miles (even if their most unpleasant memories from childhood involved gym class and running)—or trying to run. They were running to forge and solidify an identity, as Sarah does. They were running because, if they didn't, they'd rarely have social interaction with anybody older than five. They were running to find peace with their new normal of diapers or divorce. They were running so they didn't lose themselves somewhere in a pile of laundry or a pot of mac and cheese. They were running to make their days feel a little less challenging and heavy, as Dimity does. That sounds more depressing than it should, but let's be honest: Motherhood, no matter how old your kids are, is not the easiest thing ever. (That's a direct quote from Dimity's mom, so it must be true, right?)

As we collectively searched for some fresh equilibrium via pavement pounding, mother runners quickly jumped in for advice and validation. At first the questions were mostly about running: "What's a negative split, and how do I get one?" Then they became a little more casual: "I only like to wear pink tops and black capris: Is that strange?" And more personal: "I can't stand one woman in our running group who talks constantly about how great her kids are. Please advise." Finally, it got to the point where a troubling question about an unsupportive spouse or a valid concern about finishing last in a race were the norm, not the exception.

Of course, more practical questions about the best half-marathon for a girlfriends' getaway and how to treat plantar fasciitis often outnumber the more personal posts, but that's neither here nor there. Because, as we've learned during the past five years, it's the asker's point of view that really matters, and it unites us in powerful, surprisingly intimate ways. Somebody's main question may be about when to step up from a 10K to a half-marathon, but her PS may mention her son is having trouble making the adjustment to middle school or her mom has just been diagnosed with Alzheimer's or her husband recently lost his job. Even if we've never been in that situation, we all know exactly where she's coming from. Despite the speed bumps life is throwing at her, she realizes the transformative power of a mile, the importance of pushing toward new challenges, the value in taking care of herself, one step at a time. You may never meet her in person, but you know her better than you may know your cousin or cube-mate.

Tales from Another Mother Runner celebrates that connection and this community. Instead of us writing every chapter, we reached out to a variety of mother-runner writers and asked them to share tales of their miles, victories, trials, and histories. Not surprisingly, they delivered as only

BAMRs can: With wit and perspective, honesty and depth. "While [my family] supports me," writes Bethany Meyer in a piece about hiring a coach, "Training with Coach was like having my own little cheerleader who is not rooting for me and, in the next breath, asking for a ham sandwich. And there is something to be said for encouragement that comes sans a request for deli meat."

Whether you're restarting your commitment to running (again), as Nicole Knepper talks about; or ready to become an ultra-BAMR, as Katie Arnold details; or looking for joy at the track, where Kristin Armstrong unexpectedly found it; or marveling that you, a non-runner for as long as you can remember, can now tackle double digits, as Adrienne Martini does, these essays will transport you into their shoes—and fire you up to lace up your own.

The essayists are far from the only stars in these pages, though. Once again, hundreds of you took your (valuable) time filling out obnoxiously long surveys about your running and your lives, and we're so grateful you did. We've included your thoughtful responses in various forms, including "Take It from a Mother" columns, "My Running Path" narratives, "What a Mother Runner Looks Like," and "In Her Shoes." With your expert, honest help, we've hit on everything from how it feels to run a naked 5K to how hard you've ever pushed yourself in a race.

Just as there's always another mile to run, there's always another story to tell; we hope you'll continue to share them with us. You can track us down and spill whatever you want at anothermotherrunner.com (or motherrunnerstore.com, if you need a BAMR tank); Run Like a Mother: The Book on Facebook; the Another Mother Runner podcast on iTunes; @TheMotherRunner on Twitter and Instagram; and at runmother@gmail.com. We can't wait to hear from you.

Happy reading—and many more happy miles.

XO—Dimity + Sarah

01

OWNERSHIP:
You Are a Runner

"I vividly recall my first mile I ever ran: age
thirty-nine, I was unhealthy, unfit, tired, and
too young to feel that was an acceptable
way to enter another decade of my life. I
arrived at a stop sign, my one-mile marker,
feeling like I had just run 10 miles. But I
also felt like I may actually be able to run
for an entire 10 miles one day. Euphoria."

—MELISSA

TAKING THE TITLE AND RUNNING WITH IT
by Nicole Blades

The moment I knew I was a runner had nothing to do with miles or meters, pace or a race. It wasn't about a clever catchphrase on a tech T-shirt, nor was it linked to a righteous cause or campaign. Actually, my transition from nonchalant foot-shuffler "just getting fresh air" to focused road hound came down to one single word—which is fitting, I suppose, for a writer.

I became a runner the day I took high offense to being called a jogger.

I mean, a *jogger?* How dare you, madam?

My doctor committed the grand misstep during my physical almost five years ago. We were going through the usual series of health questions: alcohol consumption, caffeine, diet, sleep, exercise. The first two were easy. Zip. I've always been a lightweight when it comes to alcohol, and coffee never was a friend of mine. Plus, I was a new mother then, still nursing my fresh-from-the-oven cinnamon bun, so the no-wine-or-cappuccinos life worked well for me. The diet was on point; breastfeeding will do that for you. On the topic of sleep, we may have just looked at each other and belly-laughed. (Show me a baby who considers your sleep needs, and I'll show you right off the set of *that* movie.) When we got around to my doctor asking what I was doing for exercise, I started in with my usual, noncommittal bit: "sometimes . . . head out . . . fresh air . . . short runs . . . nothing major . . . ran a couple of races before the baby . . . these days . . . fresh air."

The doctor jotted down a note in my file and looked up at me. "So you're an occasional jogger," she said, nodding. "Do you jog on a treadmill usually, or do you go jogging outside, weather permitting?"

What I heard was, "So you're a jogging jogger who jogs to jogger jogging." Gnashing my teeth was the only thing I could do to refrain from jumping off the cold examination table—flimsy paper gown and all—to stuff cotton balls in her mouth.

Okay. Maybe I was a tad overtired, too, but the whole jogger thing just rubbed me the wrong way. It sounded lukewarm and lethargic, and I knew what I was doing out there—pounding uneven pavement, confronting plantar fasciitis, pushing through long after my music stopped and my motivation fizzled—was not even a little bit related to laziness.

My visceral, at-that-moment reaction: I am a *runner,* thank you very much, Doc.

Granted, it's just language, a noun, but there's a sensibility and community attached to the term *runner* that elevates it beyond simply being a word, giving it more meaning and rendering it part of an identity. I knew that. Still, on the ride home, I doubted myself, even though I was so confident in the doctor's office. I had always been athletic, playing sports in high school. Now as a full adult, unattached to any team, declaring I was a runner somehow made me self-conscious, unsure.

I knew I wasn't a jogger, but was I a runner? It was almost as though I was nervous about being called out, brought to the front of the room to prove my claim. (Sidebar: How would one go about doing that? *Jeopardy*, the runners' edition. . . . *What is a* fartlek, *Alex*?)

My running journey began simply enough: Living in Brooklyn, New York, I wanted to get some exercise that didn't involve staring slack-jawed at the beige walls of the local, dingy gym. I also didn't want to go to war with my wallet to pay for the latest fitness trend. Grabbing some running shoes and tights sounded like the right level of commitment for me at the time. So, jogging it was. (I know. The cruddy *J* word. But that's kind of what I was doing back then.)

A coworker told me about some "fun" races—5Ks, mainly—I should consider joining. And they were fun, for the most part. Some were set to live bands playing '80s hits along the route. Other races had things like hot cocoa or cupcakes as payoff for crossing the finish line. Soon, I moved up to longer distances (10Ks, half-marathons) where the prizes were far less sugary, but still sweet: I finished!

By the end of that year, I had an impressive short stack of race-day T-shirts and a collection of shiny medals strung with colorful ribbon. However, I still didn't feel all the way comfortable calling myself a runner. I did fun runs. I went for runs. I even found a running buddy on Craigslist. But I wasn't a *runner*. "Not a real one," said the compact critic who rented space at the back of my brain. (Don't worry: The eviction notice was served long ago.)

Stepping up to a title, grabbing it tight, and running with it may come easy for some. Others, like me, need time for the thing to set in, spread out, and grow into a natural second skin. For example, being a writer. This took time, years. In the third grade, my favorite teacher, Mr. Polka, encouraged my storytelling. He was big on creative writing, and I loved him for it. He also played Beatles records in class and didn't believe in homework, so there's that, too. I continued crafting tales in my thin, four-pack of Hilroy notebooks until I started writing for my university's newspaper. I was double majoring in mass communications and psychology; I didn't quite own the writer title yet. A story about black hair politics—my first "real" one—got a good response, and the writer career option started percolating in my head.

Ten years after I listened to "Yesterday" in Mr. Polka's class, I got paid in money—not compliments—for a story I wrote and was truly able to fold *writer* into my self-description. Although the passion was always there, the payment, and a byline in an actual, on-the-stands magazine, helped to distill it into clear confidence; the kind that develops from doing something every day, failing often, but repositioning and doing it all over again, until you get to the point where you say, *Of course I'm a writer. I'm writing.*

A similar evolution happened when I became a mother, although it's more thrilling and terrifying and less self-centered. One day, I was just me, my own person. The next day, I became someone else's person, their guide and primary influence. Overwhelmed, I read everything, I judged myself too harshly and quickly, and I copied others who seemed to be doing it better. Something about this monumental transformation didn't feel right or natural quite yet. I needed to settle into this new mode, move around in this fine, fresh suit until the seams laid flat along my shoulders and against my back, and things didn't feel so stiff.

When my now five-year-old son was seven months, we began sleep training him. After reading a few passages in two "sleep expert" books and talking to our son's pediatrician, my husband and I decided to go with the cry-it-out method. We were going cold turkey: Putting our son in his crib, kissing him goodnight, turning around, and leaving the room, ignoring any subsequent bawling or screeching until he self-soothed or cried himself to sleep.

It was rough. I vacillated between curling up in a ball in our bed with a blanket tossed over my head and threatening—then bargaining with—my husband about breaking the baby out of sleep jail. (*Sleep. Jail.* Words I actually used.) I tried to distract myself, listening to blaring music on my iPod and headphones, even taking a walk in the nippy Brooklyn streets at 1 a.m. But there was something not sitting right with me; something about my son's crying that felt off. I convinced my husband to turn on the video monitor so I could take a quick look.

"I think he's stuck," I said, my tone calm and even.

Our little boy was basically bobbing in and out of sleep while standing up, leaned against the crib's headboard. He was unable and unaware of how to bend his little knees to set himself back down. I watched on the black-and-white monitor as my husband went into the baby's room, picked up the little puffalump and gently laid him down in the crib. The child was asleep again before his father cleared the room.

Even in my frazzled state, that night was like seeing my story on the newsstands. I realized my instincts were sharp, and I really did know what to do, even when I didn't know exactly what to do. *Of course I'm a mother.*

And then there are times when it's not my eyes or my gut telling me something is real, but rather it's me actually saying it out loud, speaking it into being, that allows me to grab hold of it as truth. For me, that moment was during a freezing winter race in Central Park.

Post-birth, post-doctor's appointment, I had agreed, reluctantly, to compete in the December event after my running partner—we'll call him Ray—convinced me to enter. Ray was a road-running pro with countless races under his singlet. He was spindly and anxious and super fast. Ray could run a sub-7-minute mile, barely sweating. He was also constantly passing gas while sprinting, too. Gross, yes, but he was totally shameless about it. Ray was the runner I found through Craigslist; I wanted to up my running game after having a baby. I figured having someone experienced to motivate and hold me accountable would help this mama stay on track.

And it did. I mean, I entered a bloody 10K race in the middle of a brutal winter, dammit! Committing to this race also meant training—i.e., using magazine tips and Ray's advice—and running in the snowy streets and frosted paths of my local park. I got out there when I could, and didn't bludgeon myself with the Delinquent Stick when I couldn't.

On race morning, it was extra cold and gray out. Just rude. I wanted to go back home the minute we parked the car. Ray, not one for pep talks, gave me his usual twitchy chuckle and said, "Well, we're here now. Might as well." *Might as well . . . ?*

Thanks, Ray, you gassy bastard.

I dragged regret with me all the way up to the start line. I thought, "Why do I need to do this anyway? Who am I trying to be here?" An older gentleman nudged his way up in front of me. That small, pushy move on his part somehow tapped my battery. I went from, "What am I doing?" to "Hey, buddy, what do you think *you're* doing?" Was he counting me out of the race? And was I that easy to dismiss?

A heated focus began to stir in me. The equivocating tapered off, and I thought: I'm going run this thing, because I can. Because I'm a runner. *I'm a runner.* As the announcer counted down to zero, I was no longer muttering the phrase. I was chanting it. (Still somewhat quietly—I'm not *that* girl.)

Of course I blasted by that old guy—I had to—and kept my game face on through choppy winds that made my eyes tear up. I wasn't concerned about the weather or the time or even my pace so much; I was just fixed on finishing, because at the base of it, that's why we were all there: to finish. That's what we runners do.

Each of my titles—mother, writer, runner—has been earned through sleepless nights, countless drafts, miles that never seem to end. Each is important, each a vital part of my identity. And it's when these titles roll into one another seamlessly that I am left full, content, inching up toward full-blown happy.

"Mom, are you going running today?" he asks, snuggling under my chin. I'm sitting at my desk in my home office, looking out at the giant, snow-dusted spruce tree and inhaling the sweetness from his curly hair.

"Yes, but it's cold out there," I say. "I'm just trying to prepare myself for it, for the cold, you know?"

"Yeah, I know," he says, nodding like a veteran road runner, as if he really does know. "You should put on a warm coat, Mom—and your socks."

"Thanks, sweet potato. I will."

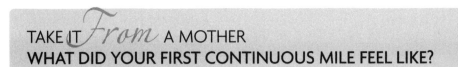

WHAT DID YOUR FIRST CONTINUOUS MILE FEEL LIKE?

"Burning, gasping elation!"

—LIESA (Set half-marathon PR less than a week after learning she was pregnant with
third baby. "I puked on some lady's shoes. Whoever you are, sorry.")

"Like my legs were heavy logs, and I was just plodding along like an idiot."

—ANN (Started running when she was sixteen. "The high school cross-country coach
needed more warm bodies, and I was lounging in the hallway after school.")

*"I was a rock star! In gym during freshman year of high
school, I finished right along with the 'athletic' kids."*

—JESSICA (Won her age group at a 5K with a 27:15. "Usually that time wouldn't be fast enough, but there
were only seven of us in my age group in a race of mostly high school kids. It was an amazing feeling!")

*"The most torturous mile of my life. I felt like my lungs were
collapsing, like my legs were revolting, and I'm certain my brain gave
up on me. But I did it, and haven't looked back ... mostly."*

—ADRIENNE (On the night before a race, called the hotel front desk at 10:45 p.m. to have them shut
down a party on her floor. "I felt like the oldest, meanest lady ever but, hey, I needed my sleep.")

*"Hopeful. I'd just been dumped, and I knew I could either
eat chocolate or get fit. I picked the latter. As I learned to redefine
myself, I was happy. I was doing something constructive for the
new me and secretly relieved the boyfriend was gone."*

—CATHRYN (Eventually ended up with a "delicious new boyfriend" who trained
with her for the London Marathon. He is now her husband.)

"Like I had conquered the world!"

—DEB (Motto: *Run Sure.* "My family is Scottish, and our clan motto is *Stand
Sure*, meaning stand with strength and confidence. So I *Run Sure*.")

"A miracle!"

—KAREN (Loves the challenge of a 10K. "Not too short, not too long.")

"Invigorating! On yucky runs, I remind myself this accomplishment was just a few years ago . . . and I remind myself how far I've come."

—ALISON (Over the years, running mentality has transformed from "Just finish" to "PR mode" to "Enjoy the moment.")

"So much fun! I ran to the hospital, which was nearby, to see my friend Jane's new baby. I didn't plan it or think it through; I just ran. However, my face gets really red when I exercise, so it was beet-red when I walked in. The nurses thought I was having some sort of emergency!"

—CYNTHIA (Can't stand sports bras that don't have a back clasp.)

"I couldn't believe how much it hurt."

—SARA (Perspective on balance: "Sometimes work wins; sometimes home wins. I've never felt like I'm winning at both at the same time—and, yes, I love to win.")

"A lifeline. My son was stillborn, and I desperately needed an outlet for my grief. For that mile, I didn't feel anything except freedom, which was everything."

—JONI ("Being on the treadmill, running as fast as my legs could carry me, made me feel as if I were one step ahead, like I could survive and outrun this pain.")

"Like a total badass. I had never run a mile, even in high school. When I finished, I jumped up and down and screamed and cheered. I looked like a total lunatic, I'm sure. Then I came in the house and high-fived my husband and two daughters."

—JAMIE (Records evening TV shows she wants to see, goes to bed early so she can run at 5 a.m., then watches shows the next evening at 7. "Running needs to fit into family life. Family life does not revolve around the run.")

I JUST TRY REALLY HARD
by Meredith Atwood

"Well, I'm not *really* a runner," I told the teeny girl—clearly a runner—at the gym. We were in the locker room. My towel was wrapped tightly around my body, making me look like a giant, white sausage. Her towel, loosely draped around her fit frame, seemed to wrap around her twice. "Yeah, not really a runner," I said again. "I just try really hard." I figured that sabotaging qualification bought me some sort of pass for my big butt and woeful treadmill pace.

I have muttered that line—*I just try really hard*—with my head hanging down, more times than I can count. Dozens of times, if not a hundred. Five words that completely disqualify my running and are completely ridiculous, considering all the *running* races I have completed. I started running in 2010, and since then, have crossed finish lines in dozens of 5Ks and 10Ks, and a handful of half-marathons. Oh, and four half-Ironman triathlons, which include, *ahem*, a 13.1-mile run.

Most ridiculous of all, I am fairly certain these laughable words escaped my mouth during the throes of training for an Ironman—a crazy distance triathlon that culminates with a marathon. Although it's likely I was at the gym, probably feeling compromised in a napkin-sized towel, I still couldn't believe what was coming out of my mouth. *Never mind that I'm going to run 26.2 miles. A runner? Oh, no. That's not really me. I just try really hard.*

About eight weeks into Ironman training, this realization finally penetrated my skin: No matter how ploddy I was plodding along on any given day, if I laced up my shoes and went for a run, I was a runner. A runner. Me. There wasn't a certain mile or *ding ding, light bulb!* moment: just the acknowledgment that I worked just as hard—if not harder—than the teeny girls, and my miles were exactly as long as the ones they covered. I began to recognize the good things that made me a runner. My sports bras and shoes were stinky, like every other runner I knew. I was chafing everywhere! *Yay! Chafe!* I needed lots of socks. I thought about running all the time. I was ticking off 8-, 9-, 11-, and 14-mile runs. Hard, long runs. And I wasn't doing myself any favors by discrediting the hard work I was putting in. (Especially because confidence is a vital ingredient for Ironman success.)

So I began to say things like, "Yes, I am training for an Ironman" and "I ran 9 miles before work this morning." I started stretching my hamstrings, unabashedly, in the checkout line at the grocery store. I spent time with a chiropractor and physical therapist for my aches—because suddenly, I was *worth* it, and so was my *running*. I took ownership of my inner athlete—specifically, my inner runner—and I began to appreciate her.

Along with ownership came some Type-A crazy momentum. I woke up earlier and earlier, and met the streets with as much of a smile as I could muster that early. *Go me! Watch me run!* I logged my miles more diligently. *Stay strong*, I'd say to myself all the time. *You are a runner!* And runners try harder. I began to think other things like, *Go faster, Meredith. You can do better than this!* Into my daily mental talks, I integrated arguably good words: Momentum. Drive. Stamina. *Get you some, mother runner!*

All good, but a new, strange little devil also entered the picture. As I sweated and strived, she sat on my shoulder and talked trash to me. *You could run faster if you would put down the cheeseburger and beer, ya know, Two Ton.*

I remember one particular day when the little devil showed up on a 14-mile treadmill run, three months before Ironman. I was at the gym, and the whole run, I heard her: *You should be running faster. Look at that girl over there. In those cute capris. And her ponytail even swishes perfectly. She looks like a gazelle. No, a cheetah. Wow, she's amazing . . . Meredith, why can't you run like her? What's wrong with you? Are you seriously ready for an* Ironman?

About 6 miles into the run, I burst into tears. Leaping off the treadmill, I tripped past the ladies on the ellipticals, the dudes doing bicep curls, and a pair doing some burpees—and ran to the bathroom, my face streaked with tears. I looked at my ugly cry-face in the mirror, and I whispered, *What are you doing? You can't do this. You are fooling yourself.*

That day, I told the pint-sized demon, who was wearing a tech tee even though she was just sitting on my shoulder, to shut the F up. I pounded out 8 more miles by myself, but it wasn't enough to make her go away permanently. She taunted me regularly, whispering comparisons to other runners and cyclists. *Look at your legs. Why don't your calves look like hers? Why can't you pedal fast enough to hang on her wheel? You really think you can finish that race in seventeen hours? It's a long road, girlfriend.* She fed this new fire inside of me—a not-so-great flame that made me somehow think I *still* wasn't good enough to be a "real" athlete. I was a runner. Okay, fine. But I still wasn't an athlete—and definitely not a *triathlete*.

You really bit off more than you can chew with an Ironman, haven't you, fat girl?

I woke up on race morning of the Ironman, and for some reason, the persistent little bugger failed to show up that day. *Phew.* I thought maybe she was finally gone, that bitch of a trash-talking naysayer. On that beautiful, perfectly perfect Sunday in June, I finished a pretty fast 2.4-mile swim, a painful 112 miles on the bike, and a very introspective marathon, where I (re)learned so many things about myself. *I have an amazing family. I am blessed beyond words or space or time.*

I am tough and strong and amazing, but these porta-potties are disgusting. I want a cookie. Pizza. Beer. Mmmm, beer. Oh, the finish line! Hallelujah!

At the finish, I was on top of the world. I did it! I met the big goal, bought the overpriced "I did it" gear, and got the signature M-DOT tattoo on my ankle to broadcast to the world not only was I a runner, but also a cyclist, a swimmer, and an Ironman, too.

Crisis solved, right?

Wrong.

Apparently, I was showing off and telling the whole world I was an athlete. But I still hadn't owned it *myself.* The little devil, not yet defeated, was hovering, lurking for another "in," another way to restart the relentless torment.

In the weeks and months following the race, I found myself thinking, *Wow, if only I had been faster. If I had not stopped to pee FIFTEEN times, then my bike time would have rocked. Why didn't I train harder? Could I have trained harder? Dammit, I regret that I didn't get the weight off my body before race day.* The whole thing was a buffet of dammits, really.

All that hard work? The 100-mile bike rides, the sunburned arms and funny tan lines, the missing toenails, and the ruined, chlorinated hair? The thousands of meters in the pool, hundreds of miles on the run and bike? Weeks of training and 140.6 miles of racing, and all I could own was my disappointment in my finishing time. When people would ask about my time, I would start to mumble. I had a new qualifier: The Ironman Edition of *I just try really hard.*

"Well, I barely finished," I would say, even though I came in 16 minutes under the seventeen-hour limit, which feels like an eternity.

I'd come back to the evil cycle. The cycle of not being a real athlete, not being a real runner. *How did that happen again?*

Immediately, I knew I had to dig out of the lunacy. I knew it was a stupid place to be, yet I didn't know how to find a route out. If I wasn't careful, I was going to find myself signing up for yet another Ironman, just to make the darn point I could be better, be a real athlete. And emphasize I was a real runner. Again.

This had to stop.

So I started doing yoga.

On one special day, I went to the 6 a.m. class. Spread out my mat. Took to *shavasana.* The room was dark (and hot), and the instructor's voice filled the air. "Meet yourself where you are. With no judgments, no expectations. Feel where you are, and be here in the moment."

What? I thought. *Love myself? Today? Where I sit, forty pounds overweight and stressed out and tired and full of issues?*

"Meet yourself where you are," the instructor repeated.

Her words made me understand what I was missing. I was trying to own Ironman and running and momentum and speed and fire, but I had no ownership of *myself*. Ownership of the awesomeness that *was* within me—right in that moment—no matter where I was. For so long, I'd focused on the races and the numbers and forgot *who* was doing the races and producing the numbers. Me. My body. That I happen to inhabit.

I'd ignored the critical component of finding grace and peace in my current athletic state, the current space in which my body existed. I'd spent so much time looking down the line at what's next, what I could accomplish, what I could do, I never bothered to slow down and meet the amazing athlete I was and praise the accomplished body I have. The amazing athlete I am today, as I sit here typing this, my thighs spread across the chair. (Thighs which happen to have run 6 miles and swim 2,500 meters before work. *Booyah!*)

Historically, I had accepted myself only with caveats. *I will get better. I will get faster. I will be thinner. When I am an Ironman, I will be a real athlete. When I am (fill in whatever), I will be happy.*

When I was lying on the yoga mat in that clammy room, I decided to buy into—and own—all of me. My athleticism, my successes, my failures, my femaleness, my strengths, my weaknesses, my thighs, my calves, my issues. All of it. I was present in the yoga class. I met my current self there and greeted her with loving arms. I did my best to hug her regularly on that day, and in the following days. I was more patient and compassionate with her. I didn't put added pressure on myself. I just was. Me.

It was hard. It's still hard. But if there's one thing I know how to do, it's how to try hard. I'm trying hard to own every cell and every bit of cellulite on my body, every inch I run, the M-DOT on my ankle, the person I have been, the person I am today. Day by day, I'm learning to love the athletic me, the triathletic me, just me, right where I am.

Six weeks after that transformative yoga class, I had one of the most powerful races of my life. The distance? Not an Ironman, but the ever-amazing 5K, the distance where most runners begin.

In January, I showed up at the race in the freezing cold with about five hundred other runners. I wore my signature, never-leave-home-without-it visor. My favorite shoes. I was the same ol' girl I've always been, but I felt more *like me* than ever. I met all of myself there. That day I told myself I was going to own this race, because I was in the perfect shape to do just that.

From the sound of the starting buzzer, I was gone. My feet turned over fast and lightly. My form was strong. My quads were burning but powerful, and I could feel them being team players. Eminem was loud in my ears, my breathing like a freight train. At the turnaround, I slowed significantly, and I didn't think I would be able to finish with the pace I had hoped. But for some reason, I came back—and I found myself again. The rhythm returned, and I powered through. Left. Right. Power. Strength. Life. Breath. Left. Right. Left. Right. I. Am. A. Runner.

During the race, not one time did a negative thought come rushing through my head. There was no chatter of, "Wow, you are slow" or, "Shake that moneymaker, big girl." Often during a race, I cannot get past the feeling of inadequacy as I am passed by eight-year-old boys or eighty-nine-year-old ladies. I cannot stop thinking about the jiggling that's happening on my thighs. Usually I am out there running with all sorts of yuck going on between my ears.

As I crossed the finish line with a solid new PR, I felt alive. I felt whole. I felt *like me*. I was proud of myself. I was proud of the personal record, of course. But I was proudest of something else.

Despite owning a tech tee, the snarky demon didn't show up. I couldn't hear her as the crowd rumbled around the starting line. I couldn't hear her heckling me as the kids ran past me. I couldn't hear her commenting on my bum jiggle. I could not hear her at all. But I could hear *something*.

In my head, I heard another voice, a different voice. Boy, she was loud. She was screaming, "Run, baby, run!" and "Nice pace, keep it up." A new, fresh, vibrant voice. The inner devil was quiet, because this new voice—the runner, athlete, person I am today—was incredibly loud, extremely victorious.

For 29 minutes and change, my cheerleader was all I could hear. After the race, I hugged her and myself.

TAKE IT *From* A MOTHER
WHAT ABOUT RUNNING MAKES YOU SMILE?

"Downhills, good music, snowflakes."

—MEGAN (Sings "My thighs are on fire" to the tune of Alicia Keys's "Girl on Fire.")

"Mile 3. At mile 3, I'm warmed up and something happens. I suddenly feel strong and invincible, like I could just keep running forever."

—CYNDIE (Ran track in high school, "mostly so I could run by the tennis courts and flirt with my future husband.")

"Those miles where I am faster than I expected."

—MARIANNE (Paced her brother, who recently lost ninety pounds, to a sub-30-minute 5K. "In our twenties, we drank beer to bond. Now we run races.")

"The release of the noise in my head."

—ANGELA ("I am fast. I am strong," is written on her Road ID. "I'm sure if I'm ever found in a ditch somewhere, the person who finds me is going to be impressed with that one.")

"I admit it: the gear. I love the cute shoes and shirts and hunting for the perfect shoe pod or iPhone armband."

—JULIANA (Working on her mental toughness. "There are many times when I'm tempted to stop because it's 'hard,' but my legs are fine and my lungs are fine. I just have to push through the doubt.")

"I love being at mile 6 and still feeling strong."

—JULIE (Completed a 13-mile training run while pushing her forty-pound son in the stroller. "He yelled at squirrels the whole way. Proud of him for holding it together.")

"The freedom I feel with each pounding step."

—ANDREA (Needed to stop at every porta-potty during St. George Marathon so "I didn't crap myself. Seriously, did I just write that?")

"Running on a sunny day."

—AUTUMN (Lives in northwest Pennsylvania, where she can go weeks without seeing the sun. "Yes, weeks!")

"Um, being done? Also, burgers."

—KATIE (Also: running through Wisconsin winters. "Totally badass.")

"Seeing goats on my run, which cheer me up for some reason.
I also love shirts with thumb holes and fold-over cuffs."

—KRISTIN (First mile of running: "Dear God in heaven, make it stop.")

"The random signs along race courses, like SMILE IF YOU ARE NOT
WEARING UNDERWEAR. How can you not love that?"

—MARISSA (Chanted "prayer, practice, patience, perseverance" through her first 5K.)

"Making it up a long, steady hill without stopping because I
know I'll get a break when I go down the other side."

—JODIE (Started running because her kids were driving her nuts. "I made it down the block and thought, 'Huh. I could probably do this on a regular basis.'")

"The accomplished feeling that goes with hobbling around after a hard run or race."

—CARLY (Tagline for 2014: "Be brave enough to bet on you." —Kara Goucher)

"Whenever a BRF I am running with says, 'I have a
story that's going to take a mile or two.'"

—KAREN (Admits her upper body is weak. "Do I really need it as a runner?")

"Uninterrupted time that doesn't involve multitasking."

—VANESSA (Would tell beginners to "ignore the folks who say you 'have' to do anything. Listen to your body instead.")

"I love feeling like part of a great, big, universal group of runners. We
all share this passion for getting out there and hitting the pavement,
which not everyone—including much of my family—understands."

—DIANE (Her "super-sore boobs" during pregnancy forced her to stop running.)

BABY BUMP AND RUN
by Jenny Everett

In the waiting room before my six-week postpartum check-up, I jotted down questions for my MD: Is the hard lump in my left boob a clogged milk duct? Can I have sex? Is it okay to start running again? Her answers: No (*phew*), yes (*yikes*), and yes (*YOWZA*). The nod to lacing up meant I could finally reclaim my body after five years of fertility treatments, pregnancy and—*huzzah*—the birth of a healthy baby boy, Sam.

Running has always given me a sense of control. When my father had his first open-heart surgery more than a decade ago, I told myself if I ran 10 miles, Dad would be okay. I did, and he was. Are the outcomes even remotely related? Nope. But mentally, it did the trick. The run-it-out approach also worked for overcoming the death of pets, job layoffs, and breakups with douchey dudes who seemed dreamy at the time.

In 2008, when my husband, Dave, and I started trying for a baby a few months after walking down the aisle, I was running five days a week. I felt very much in control. I had just completed my first half-marathon. My body was ready for this. I figured just as I'd trained for and completed the race, we'd simply *get pregnant*. I mean, given the number of oops-I-made-a-baby-and-didn't-even-know-it-till-I-went-to-the-ladies-room-at-my-prom TV reality shows, it can't be that difficult.

Apparently, I would not be a good cast member in said programs.

After a year without success, we calmly made an appointment with a reproductive endocrinologist who did some tests and told us my tubes and uterus were palatial and Dave's sperm count and motility were excellent. Go home and have a lot of sex for six months, he prescribed. (Insert eyebrow raise from the delighted husband.) For months, we lived and romped according to ovulation tests. If I got smiley face in the stick's window, Dave hurried home from work for Project Baby action. I spent the rest of my time trying to optimize my baby-making hormones: I ran regularly (carefully tracking my heart rate so I wouldn't push too hard), did lots of supported shoulder stands to "open my womb" and to balance my girly chemistry, went to acupuncture twice a week, and ate the fertility-friendly organic foods prescribed by books and bloggers. (Including the repulsive core of a pineapple, which aids with implantation, I had read.)

But month after month, Clearblue Easy (easy, my ass!) reported we were decidedly not pregnant. I went from frustrated to panicked. So back to the fertility doctor we went, where I was officially stamped with the "unexplained infertility" label and started on treatments.

I remember exactly where I was standing—in the middle of a coffee shop, in my bathroom, at the counter at J. Crew, at the corner of Meeting and Broad streets with dog leash in hand—when I got each call that our three intrauterine inseminations (think: turkey baster) and one round of in vitro fertilization (surgically removing the egg and fertilizing it outside the womb) hadn't worked. Each time, I swallowed back tears and called my husband and told him those particular eggs and sperm just weren't meant to be our baby.

Then I did what I always do when hardship strikes: I went for a run, and wondered what the hundreds of injections of Follistim and progesterone and Lupron were doing to my body. *Maybe it's not worth it. Maybe my 5' 1" frame isn't capable of carrying a kid. Maybe I'm just not meant to be a mom.* But by the end of the run, I'd convince myself to try again. *We will have a baby.*

Of course, I also remember where I was standing when the Coastal Fertility Center called to say our second round of IVF had worked: in my kitchen, sipping a cup of decaf green tea. The phone number flashed on my screen, and I braced for the gut punch. "Hi, Jennifer. It's Andrea. How are you?" *Okay, enough small talk. Cut to it.* "You're pregnant." *Omigod. This is happening. There's a baby in my uterus. Holy crud.* Everything was different in that instant.

Pregnancy was pretty easy on me. I didn't gain a ton of weight, and even managed to continue running—though inconsistently—into my seventh month. I knew my first post-baby run would be hard, but I had faith I'd retained some muscle memory and endurance. After all, hours of pacing with a swaddled newborn certainly felt like interval training. I was cautiously optimistic I wouldn't feel absolutely terrible. Physically, anyway. Mentally: another story. The one and only time I was away from my nugget in the first six weeks was a quick trip to the grocery store. Sam screamed the entire time. "Jenny, this is DEFCON 1; I need backup," my husband attempted to yell over Sam when he called me. Standing in the checkout line, paging through *People* magazine, I felt overcome with guilt. *My kid needs me, and I'm reading about Prince George.*

With that moment needling my memory, I had strategically timed a run so Sam was freshly nursed and had dozed off. "Just topped him off," I reported to Dave as I nervously fiddled with the drawstring on my shorts. *Hmph.* No need to tighten that sucker. After making a backup bottle just in case Sam decided to replay the grocery-store meltdown, I layered on two sports bras for two reasons: so my newly acquired cleavage wouldn't bounce around and to avoid any unsightly leakage.

I assured Dave this run would be extremely short. "Thirty minutes, max," I promised as I laced up my Asics and walked out of the house with that feeling you get when you just *know* you are forgetting something: your wallet, keys, phone—a, umm, 8.5-pound human. No car seat. No burp cloths. No swaddle blankets or diaper-blowout backup outfits. I felt weightless, though I knew that would change upon taking my first few postnatal strides.

I had absolutely no plan, except to run until I was tired and sweaty. No route. No set pace. No mileage goals. And only one rule: This run was about *me*. It was an escape. I could not spend the entire time thinking about Sam. *Good luck with that.*

Minute 1:00: Heading out into the ninety-degree Charleston heat, I fire up our delivery room playlist, an admittedly questionable decision given the aforementioned rule. But if it could motivate me though labor, it could certainly push me through this maiden mommy voyage. I decide to skip a warm-up—no time to waste. I take a left out of our street and head toward the waterfront to the sounds of Citizen Cope.

> *Well, a son's gonna rise in a mile*
> *In a mile*
> *You'll be feeling fine*
> *In a mile you will see*
> *After me*
> *You'll be out of the dark, yeah*
> *You'll get your shot*

I'm not thinking about Sam; instead, I'm thinking about everything that led up to him. Crazy that, a year ago, we hadn't even begun the injections for our second IVF cycle, the one that finally worked. Before starting our fertility treatments, I had pushed myself on runs. I had completed dozens of 5Ks and 10Ks and enjoyed trying to beat my personal best on loops around the Central Park reservoir in New York City, where we lived at the time. But I had stopped running hard a few years into trying to conceive. I was scared it would somehow exhaust my body and cause me to produce even crappier thirty-five-year-old eggs. After five years of trying—hundreds of injections, surgery to remove adhesions around my tubes (turned out they weren't so tidy after all), and more than $50,000 spent on treatments—I wasn't sure how much more I could take.

Minute 4:00: Running along the Charleston Harbor, I think about the routine I had had: After every appointment with our reproductive endocrinologist, no matter how good or bad the news, I had taken our Boykin spaniel, Pritchard, for a walk to clear my mind. I so badly wanted to be a mom. I wanted to know what we would get when we put together my dark complexion with my husband's wavy red hair and bright blue eyes. After we were engaged, Dave once said, "We are going to have the coolest kid." It was a sweet, out-of-nowhere remark. I had wanted to show him—and myself—he was right. But families come in all different forms. *Ours will be what it's meant to be*, I had told myself. *We will be okay. We have each other.* Big exhale.

The sea breeze brings me back to the present.

I really hope Sam's not crying. Either way, he'll survive. Right? Right. Well, I hope Dave isn't too stressed. Oh, great, my right boob is already leaking. *Just sweat, people. Nothing to see here.*

Minute 6:00: The air is sticky and hot, and I'm starting to get a feel for my new mom-ified body. My gait feels different, as though my legs don't quite line up beneath my hips, and my belly jiggles. I should've worn three sports bras. I'm already tired. Have I even gone a half mile? Labor was easier than this. At least we were cut a break on that end of the baby-making deal. Epidural before induction = best idea ever.

Minute 10:18: As I turn to head north on the peninsula, I hit my stride and realize my body can still do this. The Adidas MyCoach app chimes in to announce I've covered a mile in 10 minutes, 18 seconds. Could be worse.

While forty-five-day-old Sam's style trends toward graphic tees, cargo pants, and tiny Toms, when I left the house he was wearing an "I was worth the wait" onesie. It was an Etsy find I'd been eager to put him in since I bought it, just after we cleared the first trimester. My best guess is he's now farting in his sleep, occasionally flashing a crooked sleepy smirk. When I inhale, I can smell his eau-de-lavender-lotion-and-spit-up wafting off my left shoulder.

Minute 15:00: I pass a mom running with one of those BOB strollers. I've told myself running would remain a *sans*-baby escape: just me and the pavement, like back in the day when I'd sprint along with the other 6 a.m. Central Park regulars. We'd nod in acknowledgment, but we were relatively alone in a big, crazy city.

Fat chance, I think. *You gave up solitude the minute that catheter was inserted into your uterus to deposit a five-day-old cluster of blossoming cells.* Maybe I should just get the stroller.

Besides, if I'm being honest, I hate being away from Sam. Ever.

Minute 21:00: Circling a lake near our house, my joints start their protest, which is convenient because I'm pretty much dying to get home and see my red-headed boy and red-headed husband.

I always imagined my kid with dark hair and eyes like I have. But Sam looks just like his daddy: strawberry hair, striking blue eyes, and skin that will require SPF four million. The paternal resemblance delights me. I can't wait to see them in a few years, with matching mops of red hair, reeling in fish in the Charleston Harbor.

Minute 26:00: My heart races as I turn into the narrow alley where we live. I'm not really exhausted, but welling with emotion. Tears mix with sweat, and I realize this is the first time I've allowed myself to cry since Sam was born. Maybe I had been afraid to truly acknowledge his existence in such a visceral way because it may not actually be real.

I still can't believe he's mine. That I'll walk in the door, and my son will be there. *My son.* After all of the poking and prodding, hope and heartbreak, he's here.

As Mumford & Sons play through my earbuds, I decide to do an extra lap around the block so Dave won't be able to tell I've been crying.

> *Well, I came home*
> *Like a stone*
> *And I fell heavy into your arms*
> *These days of dust*
> *Which we've known*
> *Will blow away with this new sun*
>
> *But I'll kneel down,*
> *Wait for now*
> *And I'll kneel down,*
> *Know my ground*
>
> *And I will wait, I will wait for you*

I walk into a quiet house. Pritchard, our four-legged baby, greets me, per usual, with a wiggling brown butt. "Hi, Mama," Dave whispers. "Did you think about Sam the entire time?"

"Hardly at all," I say. He knows I'm lying.

Sam, of course, slept the whole time.

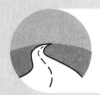

MY RUNNING PATH

"I want *stories*," writes Clover, a mother runner of two in Portland, Oregon. "I love my running friends, but their talk of numbers and paces and GPS's and age-graded blah-blah-blah absolutely bores me senseless. I love a good race report, but no numbers please. Well, except for your finishing time. I want to know that."

Roger that, Clover. We love a good race report, too, but the best kind of mother-runner tales? Birth stories. Not the "I was in labor for twenty-seven hours and pushed for five more" kind, but the "Why I finally decided to run a mile" version.

So here's a smattering of getting-started stories:

In 2009, I was watching Meb Keflezighi running away in the New York City Marathon, and I had this almost primal urge to run. I stood up in my living room and "ran" the last mile of the marathon along with Meb. The running itch stayed with me for the next year, although I did nothing to scratch it. I always had an excuse: no shoes, no sports bra, I'm too old, I'm not athletic, etcetera.

In the summer of 2011, I bought a tech shirt to run in. I looked at it for a few months. Fall of 2011, I volunteered to work at the New York City Marathon. I distributed bib numbers at the expo, which was indescribably fulfilling. Two days later, as I was handing out Mylar blankets at the marathon finish line, two events occurred that finally got me moving. First, I saw an Achilles athlete with two prosthetic legs cross the finish line. I said to myself, "Kathleen, if that man can run 26.2 miles without two legs, you can run 1 mile with two good ones." Second, as a young woman crossed the finish line, she was weeping uncontrollably. "Are you okay?" I asked, "Do you need medical attention?"

She said, "I just need my mom."

I said: "I'm a mom. Will I do for now?" She threw her arms around me. I hugged her for a few minutes and told her what an amazing person she was and that she should be proud of her accomplishment.

The next day I started the Couch to 5K program. I've been running ever since.

—KATHLEEN (Her large chest doesn't allow her to wear cute racer-back tank tops. "When I do, I feel like my boobs are going to bounce off my body . . . although I wish they would, because then I could wear cute racer-back tank tops.")

In my twenties I was lean, strong, loved life, and loved to run. I was pretty fast, and often placed in my age group. I ran a marathon in 4:01. I had my son at age twenty-seven, and then my husband left us. I was in a new city, no job, no friends, no family nearby. I fell into a deep depression that required multiple hospitalizations, began to drink much too heavily, and stopped all forms of exercise. I spent my thirties just surviving life. I quit drinking, got a teaching job, started therapy and medications.

When I turned forty, I started running again. But I didn't stick with it: lots of starts and stops. A few years later, I went to hear a female triathlete and coach give a talk on healthy life choices and motivation. I hired her on the spot, and she has been coaching me ever since.

I'm not as fast as I was in my first running life, but at age forty-seven, I'm faster than I was four years ago, when I finished a half-marathon in 3:20. My goal for 2013 was to break three hours—and I did it twice!

I've had to rethink what it means to be an athlete because my size and speed have changed significantly since my twenties. But I am strong, and I am reshaping my body and mind. And once again, I love life.

—CAROL (Goal for her fiftieth year: Run a marathon. "And I have a secret goal of completing a half-Ironman triathlon one day.")

When I was thirty-five and the mom of four kids, my sister said, "Hey, let's run the Disneyland Half-Marathon." I agreed. The race was amazing. I cried as we ran through Angel Stadium. All these people were cheering my name—it was on the bib!—and I thought, I have a ten-month-old baby and three other kids at home! This is the first time in my life I've had to work this hard to accomplish a goal.

I can't describe the happiness I felt then, but you're runners: You get it.

—JESSICA (On every run, she needs to hear Eminem's "Lose Yourself.")

I was required to take a running class in college. Although the first few weeks were hard, I continued to run when it was over. For a long time—through getting married and having three kids—I ran 3 miles, four or five times a week. The only time I didn't run was when I was pregnant.

I never raced, though. I loved the feeling I got from running so much; I didn't want to burn out. I was a competitive swimmer, and I knew if I raced, I would get too competitive. Even so, in the summer in 2009, I had a major hip injury. I needed extended rest, and didn't run for a year.

As I was healing, my marriage started crumbling, and some ghosts I had refused to acknowledge from my past finally got the best of me. When I was nineteen, I witnessed and subsequently rescued my dad from multiple suicide attempts; PTSD hunted me down, and it nearly destroyed me. I began intensive counseling to work on myself and my marriage.

About a year later, in the throes of soul searching, my hip finally agreed it was time to run again. The first mile back on a hot August morning was glorious. It was the first time in nearly a year I smiled a true smile.

Slowly, I rebuilt my mileage and pace. Each time I ran, I found another fragment of my shattered self. I sobbed through runs some days, I raged through others, and sometimes, I was so lost in the peace of the miles, I didn't even remember my route.

I became a stronger runner, and found a stronger soul as well. I realized the things that happened to me are not my story. They are just part of my life's journey.

Since that day four years ago when I stepped backed on the road, I found power. I found a voice. I found myself. I now run races because they challenge me and teach me I am stronger than any obstacle in my way.

More important, my marriage is still intact and growing, and so am I.

—CLEARY (First marathon time: a blazing 3:31:32, using the, ahem, *Train Like a Mother* Marathon: Own It plan)

I walked for years, smoking cigarettes along the way. Then, when I was about thirty years old, walking turned into running. Turns out, it's really hard to smoke and run. I finally gave up cigarettes and never looked back.

—DEBI (Proudest running moment: finishing her first marathon in 2013. "My stepdaughter was my coach. Made it even sweeter. XO.")

I homeschool my five kids, and even though I chase them all day, I started feeling guilty about my lack of consistent exercise. I hate the heat, so I waited until the end of September to start the Couch to 5K program. The weather was perfect and so was my attitude ... until I started my first 60-second running interval. My lungs were heaving, trying to catch a breath. "Mama, this is easy," said my daughter, who was running beside me. "It's not easy for me, so be quiet!" I snapped back.

Determined not to quit, I finished the first week but ended up switching to a program that built up to running more gradually. It gave me tremendous confidence to gain endurance without the accompanying frustration.

Sometime in December, I found out about a 2-mile race and signed up. It was the kick I needed to push past my fears and start running without walk breaks; at that point, it was all mental. Once I broke through that barrier, I was on fire. Six months after starting, I ran my first 5K, then nearly a year to the day after I began running, I ran my third 5K in under 30 minutes. My eyes welled up as I crossed the finish line.

Six weeks later, I finished one in 27:33. I'm still living off that high.

—KRISTIN ("Hate to admit this, but a cream-filled chocolate doughnut is my go-to race breakfast.")

I started running after my husband bought himself a treadmill; he swore it was just what he needed to get in shape. After spending a couple of hours putting the darn thing together, then watching it sit idle for a few weeks, I decided to motivate him by showing him how easy it was to use. It took a long time, but he finally started to use it periodically. I, on the other hand, developed an addiction.

—LAUREN (Also addicted to training plans, charts, and stickers. "Never, ever forget the stickers.")

After college, I moved to New York City and needed to lose the weight I gained living the academic life, so I decided to enter the New York City Marathon lottery. Ballsy, I know. The day I found out I got in, I went to Central Park, ran two loops, and convinced myself if I could run 13 miles with no training at all, I could run a marathon with proper training.

I put in a lot of miles on my own, and I did one 7- to 8-mile tempo run weekly with my roommate's boyfriend, an ex–Penn State cross-country runner. (At the time, I definitely didn't know it was called a tempo run.) I ran 3:46, my fastest marathon of three to date.

—STEPHANIE (Best piece of race advice: "Pace yourself at the beginning. For every second you go out too fast, you'll pay at least double for it toward the end.")

As a ROTC college student I ran with the cadets, who would always leave me behind. I secretly wanted to run with bus money and jump on the bus back to campus without anybody knowing. I never did it, though. I pushed through the pain and continued to run a slow 2 to 3 miles several times a week for the next ten years. I ran through all three of my pregnancies at a snail's pace, and enjoyed the time to myself with the wind in my face.

In my late thirties, I began running to help relieve some of the stress of being a dual military couple. There's just so much time apart for numerous deployments. I used running as an escape, and for the first time, I actually wanted to run every day. And not just 2 or 3 miles, but 6 to 10 miles. Not surprisingly, I got faster. The more I ran, the more I wanted to run. And not just run, but run well.

Two years ago, I was notified I was going to deploy to Afghanistan. I knew my daughters would be cared for in my absence, so my first thought was, "Where am I going to run?" Luckily, I wasn't banished to a year of treadmill running. I was able to run outside in Afghanistan. We arrived a week before Thanksgiving, so I hung a flyer in the hallway of the field hospital for a Thanksgiving Day 10K. I got in trouble for scheduling an unplanned event—we needed security (of course), and water points—but about twenty-five runners showed up. After that one, I coordinated monthly 10Ks, with proper security and water.

Now that I've returned, I appreciate running on trails under trees in clear air and continue running in the good old U.S.A. even more. I like to think I will never stop.

—CHERYL (Daydreams of the day she'll have a whole day to just run, and "the house will magically clean itself.")

After running in high school and hating every minute of it, I started again in my early thirties when my sister signed my husband and me up for a 7-mile crazy trail race called The Humdinger. She said the training would be like hiking—which I love—but faster.

Since then, it's been off and on again for running. When I'm on, I love the feeling of accomplishment and strength; when I'm off, I hate how cranky I feel. I try to keep a race on my horizon so I have a training plan to follow. If I'm not signed up for anything, I only go when the Running Spirit moves me. And the Spirit doesn't talk as loud as my sofa.

—GWEN (During Rock 'n' Roll Philadelphia, her first half-marathon, she thinks she "smiled the whole 13.1 miles.")

My friend, whose running partner had recently moved away, coerced me into running. She skillfully exploited my desire to be in better shape for rock climbing by presenting running as excellent cardiovascular conditioning. Once I agreed to try it, she made me promise I'd stick with it for at least two weeks. "Because the first two weeks always suck," she explained.

Once I started to run, I progressed quickly, then plateaued hard. Initially, it was a lot of fun to see that I, lifelong nerd, could take up and enjoy an actual sport. I could keep up with other runners I admire. I could win my age group in races. I was awesome!

And I started thinking, "Wow, if I actually trained, maybe I could be really good." Yeah, but no. When I actually trained, the activity I loved became a chore, and I really never got that much better at it. I came to accept that my scattered, undisciplined approach was just fine for me. I mean, it's not like I am going to the Olympics.

—CLOVER (Favorite running quote: "The experts are always telling us to 'Listen to your body!' But if I listened to my body, I'd live on toffee pops and port wine. Don't tell me to listen to my body. . . . It's trying to turn me into a blob." —Roger Robinson, a Kiwi Masters runner and husband of marathon legend Kathrine Switzer)

My grandparents came to cheer me on at an elementary school track meet. I turned and looked back at my competition during one of my races. Afterward, my Grandpa gave me two pieces of advice I've never forgotten: Never look back, and run like a bull is chasing you. Thinking about it now, that may have been the only direct advice I got from Grandpa.

—MINDY (Would love to keep her water bottles under lock and key so nobody else in her family could use and/or lose them.)

Keep it brief? I'll try.

Was a guinea pig for a friend who was doing thesis on walking. Got bored. Decided to run a marathon. Stress fracture and plantar fasciitis stepped in. Ran anyway.

Did a few other races, including Equinox Marathon in Fairbanks, Alaska. Dropped out at the half: first day of snow, loads of ice, crawled up an icy hill on hands and knees.

Ran intermittently or not at all for ten years.

Decided to run Twin Cities Marathon (TCM) in 2006. Hot. Started too fast.

Ran intermittently or not at all for five years.

2011: Sister-in-law placed on lung transplant list; father turned seventy; I turned forty. Dad wanted to run TCM, his first, together. I acquiesced. Training helped to mentally survive sister-in-law's lung transplant and all that entailed.

We ran TCM. Dad dropped at half. I wanted to drop at 17. I didn't. Wanted to drop at 20. I didn't. At 21. Didn't. 22. Didn't.

Finished.

Barely.

Finally realized running is the only thing that keeps me balanced, sane, kind, healthy, and focused. Will never give it up.

—ALANA (Dream race: finishing the Equinox Marathon.)

I started running because walking took too long. Then it turned into an outlet I can't function without.

—LIZ (Have you lost weight because of running? "Today is not a good day to ask me that question. I really hate that you can't outrun a bad diet.")

When I was thirty-seven, a neighbor said she would run a 5K with me. I ran that race and a couple more. And then I tried running 5 miles. I was so proud of myself I bragged about it, which got me in trouble when my daughter's friend's mother suggested we run together sometime. Damn.

I had only done 5 miles once, so I blew her off. But she was persistent so I finally set a date just to get it over with . . . and we ran 6 miles! At the end, she told me how glad she was to have a running partner and mentioned we should run every Saturday. I sucked it up because I liked her, and the next thing I knew, she convinced me to sign up for a half-marathon. Yup: 13 miles, plus .1, which was either going to be the most exhilarating or lousiest tenth of a mile ever.

I ended up finding out I was pregnant with my third child about six weeks before the half-marathon, so our time slowed, but we finished. I was determined not to gain sixty-five pounds again with this pregnancy, so I kept running, and crossed the finish line of a 10K at thirty-one weeks.

After the baby was born, I was slow for a year, then refocused and did my second half-marathon. I ran up the hill I couldn't run up when I was pregnant. Everybody around me was walking, and there was a cop at the top of the hill. "Hey, you see that hill?" I asked him, "I ran the whole thing." He high-fived me.

—JAMI (Other athletic accomplishments: "I can dance in the kitchen holding any of my kids—ages eleven, ten, and one—for an entire song.")

I have asthma, and I'm accident-prone. When I first started, I convinced myself asthma prevented me from running much more than 2 or 3 miles. I used any injury possible—stubbed toe, ingrown toenail, similar "serious" injuries—to avoid running, and when I got out there, I took frequent walk breaks. When I was thirty-nine, I realized asthma and clumsiness were just excuses. Running allowed me to see I really am an athlete, even if I still can't hit the broad side of a barn with a bat.

—KATIE (How often, on a typical run, do you think about quitting? "Start to finish.")

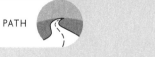

After a career change, lots of marital drama, four years of going to law school part-time while working and raising a kid, I realized I had bloomed to a shocking 210 pounds. I felt fat and out of shape. After I got my degree and my son was older, I decided to buckle down. I have never been an athlete, and never, ever a runner. In fact, I was smoking a half pack of cigarettes a day and eating a Reuben sandwich with a Pepsi most days for lunch.

A friend talked me into joining a "boot camp" fitness group, which turned out to be really laid back and led by an amazing trainer. Yet, it took me three months just to show up once. The trainer still jokes that during that first year, I said I would only show up on my birthday if we didn't have to run that day.

Somewhere along the line, though, I started to run on my own a little bit. Never too far: maybe a mile at a time. Then I started to like it and decided to quit smoking. When I wanted to reach for a cigarette, I went for a run, even if it was just to the corner and back. Once I could breathe better, I wanted to run farther and realized doing so would justify buying all the gadgets and clothes.

I ran my first 5K on Thanksgiving in 2012 and finished in 42:02. I had some foot problems that caused me to take a few months off, but after I got out of minimalist shoes and into orthotics, things improved. Six months later, I clocked a 34:07 5K and had a goal of running my first 13.1 during the 2013 Thanksgiving weekend. I battled iliotibial band syndrome for two months while training before I dropped out, and I turned my race into a vacation to Seattle instead.

I continue to struggle with my weight—I was down to 165 that summer, and I gained twenty pounds—but now I know I love to run, and I'm headed to Rock 'n' Roll Las Vegas this winter.

—KATHERINE (While running in bad weather, she realized she was "that person." And was proud.)

02

PERSPECTIVE:
A Mile Is a Mile

"When it comes to miles and times, I only compete against myself and I try to see my life more globally. I wouldn't trade my life/kids/work for really amazing numbers. I can't be awesome at everything so it's okay to try to keep my awesomeness with my kids and work—and my running can just be somewhat awesome."

—ELLEN

RUNNING FOR MY LIFE

by Nicole Knepper

When a toddler throws down the challenge, "Bet you can't catch me, Mommy," it might be because he's a competitive little punk testing boundaries. Or it might be he's desperate to get attention since you haven't responded to his last five requests to watch while he does the exact same thing—shoveling in the sandbox or something equally scintillating—he was doing the first sixteen times you actually did look.

In the case of Zachary, my firstborn, it was the latter. He wanted my attention, but he also wanted me to catch him.

But I physically couldn't.

When I was thirty-two years old and Zach was just two, he demanded every last drop of my energy. Well, he wanted what oomph I had left after I had worked all day as a clinical therapist in a therapeutic day school. Beyond working, I stole a few minutes here and there alone with my husband, and used a few more for mandatory bodily functions like eating, sleeping, and pooping, but the rest of my time was devoted to Zach.

I used that busy-working-mom excuse any time I did something half-assed or ignored something important. I let the laundry go until we all had dirty underwear turned inside out. I sent e-mail birthday greetings instead of the cards I had once so lovingly picked out, cards that had always arrived on time. The thing I *full*-ass ignored was exercise. I felt terrible about it, too, because I had been active—a regular runner, actually—all my life until I became a mother.

As if working-mom guilt wasn't gobbling enough of the precious energy I didn't have to spare, I felt guilty about not running because I knew how vital sweat sessions were to my well-being. I rationalized not running via an illogical and ongoing inner dialogue, which, even by guidelines set forth by the Society of First-Time Mothers (it's not an official membership thing, but you know as well as I do that it exists), was not up to snuff.

Guilty Me: "The baby needs me! I don't have time for me."

Healthy Me: "He's not a baby. He's two. And you can't care for him if you don't care for yourself. GO FOR A RUN!"

Guilty Me: "I'm tired. I worked all day. I need to spend time with the baby."

Healthy Me: "A run will pep you up and give you the energy you need to enjoy and extend the time you have with him. GO FOR A RUN!"

Guilty Me: "Fuck you! I'm depressed! I wish I were dead. This kid would be better off without me."

Healthy Me: "No. Fuck YOU. You know running gives you the dopamine that kicks your depression's ugly ass. You have to live to raise your son. GO FOR A RUN!"

I guess this would be a good time to address that "I wish I were dead" comment. Two full years after having my first child, I was just starting to see the light of day after suffering from a long and severe case of postpartum depression. The disease was so acute, it turned me into a suicidal skeleton.

Postpartum depression drained my body, as well as my soul. My 5' 5" frame carried only 115 pounds, and only a fraction of it was muscle. In my pre-mom, pre-depression days, I weighed a muscular, toned, energetic 130 pounds. I could knock out a 5-mile run in little more than half an hour and still have enough energy to teach or take an exercise class.

Which brings us back to the day Zach was hollering, "Chase me, Mommy!" I knew then I could catch him, but it wouldn't be easy. He was as fast and determined as I was exhausted and out of shape.

As I zigged and zagged behind Zach, I realized I'd done exactly what I'd sworn not to do: become a heart disease–courting, cigarette-smoking victim of depression. The only running I was doing was from my truth, which was this: Running was probably the only thing that could save me from the fate of my family.

Dear God, I had become my parents.

Running does not run in my family, unless you count scurrying from the law, which I understand my father did a lot of when he was in college, but that's a story for another book. What does run in my family is heart disease, and a deep history of shunning any sort of exercise that isn't directly related to avoiding prosecution, rescuing a hyperactive child in a busy street, or bolting from an angry bear in a state park—not really sure this happened, but my Uncle Ole insisted it did. Also my family is good at metaphorically running from problems and overwhelming emotions with illegal substances.

My parents grew up in homes short on cash but long on love, and one of my extended family's most beloved traditions is sitting down for a weekly, shared meal. When I was growing up, these occasions were thick with red meat, rich gravy, generous pats of butter, and plenty of salt. Before, during, and after dinner, the adults indulged in multiple cocktails and cigarettes. They sat and sat and sat some more, exercising their minds and their mouths. As working-poor immigrants, they considered a long, chatty, fatty meal to be a reward for their back-breaking work in a hard world.

I loved those Sunday dinners. The raucous laughter and good-natured ribbing fascinated me. I assumed every family spent hours at the table eating, drinking, and telling stories. Unfortunately, the first of the precious faces at the table disappeared when I was only six. My maternal grandfather died from complications of heart disease and emphysema when he was sixty-nine. Cancer took my maternal aunt and uncle within two months of each other; they left four young daughters behind. My maternal grandmother, a devoted smoker, red-meat eater, and beer drinker, died in her sleep (heart disease again). My paternal grandfather became so ill that he was unable to walk, his arteries packed with plaque from years of fat coursing through his blood. His descent was long and slow. When he finally died, it was a relief. Oh, but his laugh is the sound I miss most. It hurt to think I would never hear it again. My people were dying.

By the time I became a teenager, seventh-grade health class taught me more than I wanted to know about how my family members' habits had contributed to their deaths. I learned heart disease and emphysema didn't have to run in families. I had a choice—and so did the rest of my still-living loved ones. Like a typical kid, I nagged and whined and complained about the smoking. I smashed cartons of cigarettes and demanded my father take walks with me after dinner, but no one made any changes. How did these people who were supposed to be intelligent and responsible adults justify their behavior? They made me eat enough fiber-filled green veggies and colorful fruits to unclog the bowels of a rhinoceros, but they didn't take care of their own bodies.

In addition to my five-a-day-fruits-and-veggies lifestyle, I took a 180 from my family, activity-wise. As a kid, I was into gymnastics, ice skating, dancing, and swimming. I ran track in junior high and was an excellent hurdler. I didn't stay with running as a team sport, but I developed a love—and need—for it.

During my junior year of high school, I had my first bout with depression. Antidepressants helped, but running helped more. *I ran to feel.* Sometimes I was totally empty, and running made me feel something. Other times I was overwhelmed, and running helped lighten the load.

I was young and dumb, though, and started smoking cigarettes. I continued to light up through college, even though I was studying to get a bachelor's degree in exercise science and fitness management. (Like I said: young and dumb.)

But back to the day I couldn't catch Zach. It was a magnificent, warm spring afternoon. I was smoking good old Marlboro Reds as my son, leaping around the backyard, offered up the bait: "Come get me, Momma! You can't get me."

The kid was right. I couldn't get him. He was hauling his little diaper butt this way and that, giggling and enjoying the fact I was probably going to relent and give him more time in the yard because I kept needing to stop and catch my breath. It was awful, and I was furious. My spirit was willing, but my flesh was fried. Feeling shitty made it hard for me to keep my cool when my kid was giving me the business; each time I lost my temper, I felt even worse.

Poor kid was just doing what kids do: testing the boundaries and looking for his momma to set them. He was enforcing his right to be a terrible two-year-old. It always took a monstrous effort to round him up and get him to go inside as the sun was going down, but this night in particular, it was nearly impossible. Gasping for breath, I walked into the house with a kicking toddler under one arm. I was thirty-two years old, and I had become exactly what I didn't want to be. *How could I be too goddamn tired to make dinner?* I served a junky meal. More guilt. After his nuggets and fries, I was too weak to carry my son up the stairs. He was too tired to walk. There was a lot of whining from both of us. I still felt winded while reading him a bedtime story.

Would the shame and torture of this day ever end?

Was this how life was going to be now?

That was it. I knew I had to run again.

I won't tell you how hard it was to go from being a rail-thin, junk-food-eating, chain-smoking, depressed couch potato into a muscular, healthy-eating, nonsmoking runner. You probably already know how hard it was. I will allow it was tough to adapt to pavement pounding, healthy eating, and cigarette resisting. But I really didn't miss couch sitting, carb binging, or chain smoking.

Pffthh . . . total lie. I missed it all. It was fucking brutal.

It was also fucking worth it. Because, turns out, I had also missed running.

Four years later, I was back to working out consistently and enthusiastically and found myself pregnant with baby number two. Despite a barfy first trimester, I managed to get in regular runs and workouts. Then I was sidelined at twenty-six weeks with pre-term labor. No more exercise. This time I was prepared for the inevitable post-baby sadness, but I had no idea how I was going to deal with the mega-fat that became part of my back and ass—and arms and neck—as a result of a little more than three months on bed rest. I wasn't just fat: I was also weak, and the muscle I had rebuilt over the past four years atrophied while I lay horizontal and grew a beautiful baby girl.

I would like to tell you that I ran off the fat like a champion, that I was both a devoted runner and mother with laser-like focus and determination. That would also be a lie. I was juggling two young kids, a second postpartum depression that was less intense but depression nonetheless, and an extra twenty-five pounds, down from more than fifty I gained while spending three months flat on my back. As if that situation wasn't hard enough, I began to experience other physical discomforts, as well. I ran when I actually had the energy and the kids covered, but that was a rare occasion. My husband was working two jobs so I could stay home. I knew the miles would help me feel better, but every time I would get a rhythm going, another weird symptom would put me on the sidelines.

On and off, I would be covered in hives, the origin of which no doctor could determine. Then came debilitating fatigue and numbness in my hands and feet. It was four years before I was diagnosed with Hashimoto's thyroiditis, celiac disease, and rheumatoid arthritis. Yes, indeed, just before I turned forty, I became the poster child for autoimmune disease. Thanks, genetics!

That shit *does* run in families. Turns out, all of those things ran in mine.

It's totally unfair, if you ask me. I get my life together, and am willing to put in the miles, but my body rebels? *What the?* That said, life always feels fair to me when I'm pounding the pavement. Running is where everything makes sense. Running is where I do my best thinking, praying, loving, healing, mental blog writing, and problem solving (and grocery-list making and kicking-my-husband's-ass-off-the-sofa visualizing).

Some days, getting out there is really hard. There are times I desperately need a playlist to keep me going because arthritis pain is a nagging jerkwad of a noise. Once I get a rhythm, one of my strengths is keeping a steady pace, but good grief, I am slow. Like Internet-dial-up slow, but I don't really care. I don't run for rewards or victories or vanity. I am running for my life.

During my runs, I often wonder if my genetic disposition for the autoimmune diseases would have kicked in had I stayed consistently focused on fitness throughout my pregnancies. Would maintaining a level of consistency in my activity have served as a preventative measure? I don't regret having my beautiful babies, but I sure wish I had prioritized my own health the way I did theirs during the early years of their lives.

As the miles pass by, I wonder if I can make running—or any physical activity—run in my current family; maybe my children and their children can be spared the pain my grandparents, parents, and I experienced? Maybe my kids and grandchildren will be less prone to the cellular switch-flip that starts a body's descent into illness? Or perhaps healthy lifestyle choices will stave off the inevitable? That glimmer of hope is enough to motivate me so my lifestyle choices will encourage them.

Despite the cloud of smoke and the stomachaches that inevitably followed Sunday meals, family meals continue to be one of my most treasured memories of childhood. I find it difficult to convey the depth of my feelings for my family; I still have moments when I need to go outside and scream out my sadness and rage. The senseless and unnecessary loss of my father, who I can hardly believe has been gone for ten years, is still so painful. I honor him by carrying on our beloved dinners.

Our Sunday dinners are just a lot healthier. Our plates are full of the good fats, healthy fish, and lean meats. My kids eat greens and colorful fruits, washed down with smoothies or cold water. Unfortunately, there are fewer people than there are chairs around the table. Most of the time, it's just the four of us. Sometimes my mom or mother-in-law joins us, but even then, our Sunday dinners bear no real resemblance to the marathon mealtimes of my childhood. My mother is wasting away from heart disease, emphysema, and related dementia. Sometimes her presence at the table is comforting, but lately, as her disease progresses, it's excruciating to know her situation was entirely avoidable. It's such an odd feeling to grieve the loss of the person sitting next to you.

The whole situation makes my heart ache, but it's an ache that drives me, not a pain that is slowly killing me. It urges me to run so I will live to be at the table on a Sunday night with my grandchildren. I want to tell stories and laugh and hear all about what my kids and grandkids are doing.

I'm so excited about it, sometimes I even visualize it. When we've had our fill of satisfying, nutritious food and we still feel light and good, we'll all go outside and enjoy the night together. And when I hear the little ones say, "Bet you can't catch me, Grandma," odds are, I will.

TAKE IT *From* A MOTHER
HOW HAS YOUR RUNNING EVOLVED OVER TIME?

"I have learned the difference between good pain (I can work through it) and bad pain (I need to stop and live to run another day)."

—KATHY (During the last mile of Ironman, she had "one of the very few moments in my life where I honestly couldn't believe that me—little me—had done something so big.")

"When I started running, I was figuring so much stuff out: when to run, what to wear, how my form was, what shoes were best, etcetera. Now I just go run."

—DEIDRA (Loves her post-run buzz: "I always say I could rule the world if I ran 5 miles every morning!")

"I am less critical of myself. I now know every race will not be a PR. I used to get mad at myself when it wasn't."

—ROSEY (Ran her first marathon a month before her wedding.)

"Not everyone can run, so I registered to run for someone else and was matched with a four-year-old girl who has a disease that will prevent her from ever running. My runs are dedicated to her, and it makes me very happy."

—NICOLASA (Favorite treadmill workout: 6 mph for six minutes; 6.2 for five minutes; 6.4 for four minutes; 6.6 for three minutes; 6.8 for two minutes; 7.0 for one minute. "I'll ladder back down, and it covers almost 4 miles.")

"I have graduated from walking to walk/run to more running than walking."

—LAURA (Has reactive airway disease, so getting enough air to match the strength of her legs is her biggest challenge.)

"I totally gave up on feeling like I need to be better, faster, and stronger. I want to enjoy my runs, and run for as long as I can, as often as I can. When I was getting caught up in thinking I 'had to' be faster or I 'had to' run longer, it stopped being fun. Enough other things in my life are hard work. I want my running to be pure pleasure."

—JENNIE (When asked for her proudest running moment, she exclaimed, "OMG: that I do it! That I did it! That I even try!")

"In my first year, I figured out what worked while training for a half-marathon. By my second year, I graduated to marathons. I ran a 50K in my third year, but have been plagued by injuries and setbacks since then. I'm starting to see that years have ways of ebbing and flowing, and the most important thing is to keep lacing up the shoes and getting out there."

—KATE (Running against genetics. "Obesity, arthritis, and alcoholism run in my family, not athletic ability.")

"I started out training for a 5K. Now, I've run a few half-marathons and a marathon. A 3-mile run, which seemed pretty crazy when I began, is usually my standard distance run now. I still need to work on speed . . . maybe that's next!"

—EMILY (Loves a banana with Nutella after a long run.)

"I'm more willing to take advice. I used to think, 'Oh, I know my body better than anyone,' and while that's true, now I factor in, 'but this person knows running better than I do.'"

—KRISTIN (Thrilled when her daughter said she didn't want to do a kids' dash and ran the 5K with her instead.)

"I'm past the PR chapter. Now I run for the joy of it and, of course, the social aspects."

—MARCIA (Loves a good 5K. "They hurt, but they're where my heart is.")

"Running used to be the thing I did to not get fat. It has transformed into the thing I love to do just for me."

—LIESA (Ran the Columbus Half-Marathon while thirty weeks pregnant. "There were bathrooms every mile: a pregnant woman's dream come true.")

"As I am getting older, I have two goals: to increase distance and to still be running when I'm sixty, as I might have a chance of placing in my age group. I'm going to outlast the competition!"

—AIRLIE (Told her husband he could have her new, expensive Bose earphones if she didn't run under 50 minutes in a 10K. "I ran 47:47—and I don't think I'll ever go that fast again.")

MOTHER RUNNER REDEFINED

by Kara Douglass Thom

I am standing at the finish line—a finish line I will not cross. Instead, I am pacing a small stretch of barricaded road in order to keep warm at the Monster Dash in St. Paul, Minnesota. The late October air has officially transitioned from Indian summer to arctic blast.

My husband is running the ten-miler. Two other families have come in from out-of-town to race the half-marathon; my former running partner is among them. Combined, we have seven kids running the 5K dressed as M&M's, including my three daughters: ten-year-old twins, McKenna and Kendall, and eight-year-old Jocie Claire. All told, there are thirty thousand registered runners. And I'm not one of them.

There is a lull between the frenetic start and the finish-line mayhem. Parents struggle to entertain small children, which makes me grateful my four-year-old son is playing at a neighbor's house. We spectators talk among ourselves. We stretch our calves on the curb. Some of us (just me?) throw in a dozen or so walking lunges. Runners not racing are easy to spot like that.

For the record, I have withheld wearing any logoed athletic apparel that would announce I am a twenty-plus-year veteran runner and triathlete with hundreds of race finishes. Before marriage, before kids, I raced weekly, sometimes twice a week. Not dressing the part takes great restraint for marathoners (I've finished seven), and especially for Ironman finishers (twice for me). Still, I am dressed in my favorite Skirt Sports running tights and an all-weather Nike jacket, so I do look like a fit mom. However, I could be mistaken for one aspiring to get to all those finish lines, not someone who has already crossed them and is now mending a broken body.

I don't believe running is to blame for my injuries. Not entirely, anyway. Before two decades of running there were two decades of dancing, and I'm pretty sure the tears in my labrum (that sheath of tissue where the hip joints rotate) began on the hardwood floors of the dance studio.

Endurance racing began well enough, and I held up until my second Ironman, at which point I became familiar with chiropractic and physical therapy. I carried on with ice and ibuprofen as needed, but nothing slowed me down. Until my twin pregnancy. When you add sixty pounds to an already compromised structure, subtle weaknesses become alarmingly apparent. After that pregnancy? I was like a bridge that needed to be condemned.

Over a decade of three pregnancies and four babies, I raced short distances and did well, raking in age-group trophies from time to time. But I can't say I ever *felt* well. I have gone to every health practitioner possible to fix whatever part ailed me: hips, lower back, pubic bone, tail bone, a carousel of revolving pelvic pain.

If I wanted to avoid surgery, which I do, I needed off the carousel. Actually, I needed to get out of the damn amusement park. After ten years of athletic starts and stops, I had to give myself permission to stop projecting when I'd recover and return to the road. Getting better was always framed by how soon I could get back to running. Instead I had to take running—and anything else that caused pain—off the table entirely.

When I told this to my physical therapist, who treats runners almost exclusively, she couldn't believe what she was hearing. "Absolutely, that's the right thing to do," she said. "But I don't ever bother telling runners that because I know they'll never do it."

I would do it.

As I watch spectators mill about, ready their cameras, check watches and smartphones, I keep checking in with myself about how I feel, probing my athletic identity: *You're the only one in your clan not running; aren't you pissed? Your running partner is out there; doesn't that make you sad? Isn't this waiting around boring?* I answer "no" to myself each time. Because I don't take anti-inflammatories on a daily basis anymore. Because I don't wake up in the middle of the night with aching joints. Because I can now step out of bed in the morning and walk pain-free. My body is finally starting to feel good again. That alone is worth being on this side of the finish line.

I feel so good, I consider treating myself to an almond latte until I notice a line snaking out the coffee-shop door. I can't risk missing my kids at the finish line and losing them among the mass of costumed runners.

When the timing clock reaches 10 minutes, I imagine my girls near mile 1. I know my ten-year-old twins can run the entire 3.1 miles. McKenna, firstborn by nine minutes, is a fierce competitor and approached the event with diligent preparation. She was the only one of my daughters who braved the elements for the last scheduled training run. While I walked our puppy around the infield, she circled the track alone for 2 miles under the darkening afternoon sky, with slush pelting her face every time she headed south.

While McKenna is running her first 5K, having put in her training for an impressive debut, Kendall, her more impatient twin, loves a good finish line. This is her third 5K. She had the confidence of a veteran runner going into the race. Then again, she's a redhead, and I'll go ahead and stereotype her further by adding *fiery* redhead. That girl has enough steam to accomplish whatever she sets out to do.

I watch the lead males and females finish the 5K, and I take note of the time on the clock as it passes over my personal best at 19:58, a time I trained diligently to break twenty years later but that remained beyond reach in my forties. That last-hurrah attempt may, in fact, have been my body's proverbial last straw. My "go-to" 5K time was between 20:45 and 21:15. My first 5K time ever was 25:23. Even though I can recall those numbers easily, I promise I'm not wondering what my finish time might be if I were racing today. Even if I'd pinned on a race number, I'd be running with my girls, most likely my youngest daughter.

Jocie Claire, my other redhead, is all about the postrace party, not so much the training. (For the record, she chose to run: She always wants to keep up with her sisters and didn't want to miss any fun with her friends.) She once described a bike ride we took together as "hateable." She has many ways to express her opinion of running. On training runs, she put more energy into eye rolling, moaning, dramatic doubling over, and the question, "When is this going to be *over?*" than she did into forward motion.

I could translate those actions: "Running is hateable."

My husband and I both raced before we met; we continued racing after we married, even after having the kids, although it flatlined the summer we had three children under the age of two. Back then it wasn't so much a family affair. We were athletic people who chose to be athletic in whatever joke we called our "free time."

Our active lifestyle was slyly soaking into our young family. Our twins would put together their own hula hoop/bike/run triathlons—so when any of my kids objected to physical activity, it took me off guard.

One day when Jocie Claire was four, she put her foot down when it was time to go to gymnastics class. When I asked her why, she looked at me with her clear blue eyes and said flatly, "Because I don't like to run."

Any well-adjusted adult would know that being contrary is the life's mission of four-year-olds. But you could argue I wasn't well-adjusted, such as I was at the time with four young children, including a newborn. In my overwhelming disappointment or extreme sleep deprivation, somehow the detail that she was only four got away from me.

I took her rejection of running personally. Because her older sisters loved to run, I assumed Jocie Claire would follow right along. If one of my daughters hated running, a sport I loved down to my degenerating hips, where had I, her fitness role model, gone wrong?

With my daughters hostage in their car seats as we drove to gymnastics—I have mentally blocked out the struggle that got Jocie Claire out of the house—I launched into a diatribe on running. I told them even I have times when I don't like to run. I told them when the alarm rings at 5 a.m., I never want to go. I told them most days I'm tired and can easily talk myself out of a run. I told them although there are plenty of things we don't like doing, such as eating certain vegetables or picking up toys, we still need to do them anyway. And then I climbed right into the saddle of my high horse and told them when my run is over, I never say, "Geez, that was a colossal waste of my time." I told them I'm always happy when I *finish* running.

Once I finally shut up, I stole a glance in my rearview mirror; nothing there but wide-eyed silence.

There are moments in motherhood when you know you are being crazy and yet you can't stop yourself. This was one of those times. When I had finished having my say, my craziness crystallized in the silence and I remembered I didn't even *like* running until I was in my twenties. That was a good fifteen years away for them.

Thank goodness children are forgiving when parents are having their own growing pains. I don't think my running rant in the car scarred them. We all put it behind us. I went back to my own running routine, and I let them get back to trying whatever they wanted, from ice skating to karate. Honestly, truly, I don't care what sport they grow to love, as long as they grow into active adults.

What came in hindsight is something most parents intuitively know: The real reason Jocie Claire said she hated running was because she didn't want to leave the elaborate Littlest Pet Shop neighborhood she had constructed in her bedroom to head to gymnastics. Transitions are tough for toddlers.

Turns out, transitions are even harder for adults.

During the summer of 2012, I was within smelling distance of that twenty-year-old 5K time. For the first time ever, I had a coach to take me through my season of sprint-distance triathlon racing. I was lifting weights, doing plyometrics. I felt strong and capable. My hip ached, yes, but that wasn't new. My on-again-off-again lower-back pain was on again and feeling eerily similar to the pain I felt when I was nine-months pregnant with twins, which I most definitely wasn't. The tight left hamstring was new, but I figured that was to be expected as a Masters athlete. So I gimped along. Eye on the prize.

Then it happened. Was it a long bike ride? Box jumps? A track workout? Too much weight on that last set of squats? Who knows?

I had to cut races from my schedule. I delayed reaching my goal. But week after week I got worse, not better. By the end of October I could barely walk. Sitting was excruciating. Spasms would grip my lower back and butt so severely they made me cry. I was a woman who birthed four babies without epidurals. I thought I could deal with pain. Not this. So I made a deal with God: If I could walk pain-free, I would let the rest go. I'd feel content with what my body had already accomplished and celebrate where I am now, not somewhere I felt I should strive to be.

I am not proud that I didn't hold up my end of the deal.

That's the problem with runners and injuries. Once you feel a little bit better you can't help but "run on it." Six months later, in the spring, I had my "comeback" during the running leg of a triathlon relay: strong pace, negative splits, fast finish, perfect execution. It was one of the best runs of my life. It may very well have been the last best run of my life.

I quickly returned to suffering through my training runs. To borrow from my daughter, running became hateable.

I began to ask myself what, exactly, was I trying to rehab? Was this process all to get to the next race? There was soul searching, there were tears at the thought of never running another marathon. But I was already pained at not being able to pick up my children for hugs or piggy-back rides. I knew for sure what I wanted most was to return my body to a place of strength, stability, and health for the long run—which, sadly, meant figuratively, not literally.

To get there, I had to give up my love of twenty-plus years, the sport that provided a sense of accomplishment and propelled my self-confidence in every aspect of my life, that created an identity for me for so long, and was the foundation for my social network. As much as running gave—and continued to give—me, I knew I wanted a future without surgery, artificial hips, walkers, or wheelchairs. I want to grow old as an *active* senior citizen in the same way I want my children to grow into active adults. I just had to let go of the notion I had held for so long that I would be a badass, gray-haired senior Olympian.

This transition went about as well for me as one does for a toddler. There was resistance, defiance, outrage, sulking, and immense sadness. I walked. I hiked. I started to look forward to Pilates class, something I had long turned my nose up at because I was partial to barbells. I recommitted myself to yoga. I walked. I walked. I walked. I engaged my glutes with leg lifts and hip raises as instructed. My physical therapist assured me it wasn't the strength of my glutes that was at issue, but the lack of neurological connection. They weren't working. I had "glute amnesia." I imagined my big ol' glute muscles chillaxing with a smoke while my poor hammies and much smaller, medial glutes took on the crippling workload.

I was as committed to my recovery as I had been to an Ironman finish. I was so busy reconstructing my walking gait and learning to stand properly, I did not have the urge to run. All I wanted was my body to adopt a new way of engaging with the world. I was so focused on the nuances of biomechanics and core strength that I didn't so much as wince when my husband took off for a run. We even hosted an annual run party at our home, and I held my ground and walked, then held my head high while I drank my postrace beer.

By summer's end, a time that, in the recesses of my mind, I thought I'd start running regularly, I just kept walking. Occasionally I let myself run, but it was never a planned endeavor. Once while walking on my favorite trail, a running friend came up behind me, and I finished the route running with her so we could visit. A handful of times I would go on a walk and realize I would never make it back in time for whatever was required of me next unless I ran a little. So I did. I put on my run like a dangly pair of earrings I saved for special occasions, like when my daughters—all three of them, including the one who claims she doesn't like to run—wanted to train for a 5K.

I am standing at the finish line—a finish line I will not cross. A runner not running, and finally and truthfully at peace with that. I am witness to my young girls becoming athletes, and it's beautiful. I can see now, whether it's my legs logging the miles or not, running will always be part of my life.

McKenna and Kendall (red and blue M&M's, respectively) come through with their orange M&M friend, arms linked, smiles wide, practically floating on euphoria from the cheering crowd. A few minutes later comes Jocie Claire, her green M&M costume setting off her red hair, with the remaining candies.

I dole out hugs and high fives and approach Jocie Claire, her cheeks rosy from the chill outside and body heat inside. She is still breathing hard as she rips into the bag of candy passed out at the finish line. I brace myself for the kind of complaints she reserves only for her mom, those of side stitches and deathly fatigue. Instead, she gushes, "That was *awesome!*"

I feel her endorphins as if they're my own. And I'm overcome with happiness.

TAKE IT *From* A MOTHER
MY BIGGEST COMPLAINT ABOUT RUNNING IS _____.

"That I don't have enough time to train like I want to.
I'd need a maid and a personal trainer."

—MARY (Admits she "struggles with putting me on my to-do list.")

"I'm goal-driven, so I never really feel done. It's like a
constant uphill, and I never reach the plateau."

—MARY (In the Air Force, at a base-wide 5K, she passed a speedy male coworker. "I was proud, but it was even better when, later that day, he told everyone I had passed him.")

"Injury! Within a few months of setting some training goals for the first time, I
got plantar fasciitis and shin splints. I had to stop running, enlist a good sports
chiropractor, and restart a few times. The whole process took six months."

—MICHELE (Started running when her now eighteen-year-old had colic. "Feeling the worst stress I had ever dealt with, I pictured myself flying freely down the road: faster, faster, faster.")

"The impact. Regardless of the shoes or running style I use, my body is beginning to
feel the effect of the miles. I cannot cope with a future without being able to run."

—SIOBHAN (Adds: "I know I shouldn't clock all my miles on the road, but running around a field makes me look a bit mad.")

"The time commitment of training for a marathon. My husband
wasn't super excited about it, so our girls will have to be a bit older
before I go 26.2 again. I like him and want to keep him around."

—ERIN (Because of chafing, can't wear anything shorter than knee length on her lower half.)

"C-c-c-c-cold Michigan winters."

—BECKY (Doesn't walk on a run unless she's taking a GU or going through weird traffic or terrain.)

"Long runs with two little kids equals endless whining. I wish there was a running sitter exchange service; it's so much easier to run without a double stroller."

—ALISON (Found loading the kids in when they're a bit groggy, bringing plenty of snacks and toys, and having tasks—like counting dogs or bikes—works best.)

"Shoes are so damn expensive."

—KAREN (Favorite race is the Daytona Beach Half-Marathon: course starts at the Daytona International Speedway, goes to the beach, and ends at speedway finish line.)

"It looks so much easier than it is."

—LAURA (Advice to a runner standing on a starting line: "Pardon my French , but f*ck what everyone thinks. You've got this.")

"Used to be shin splints, but now it's the wind. It always feels like Category One Hurricane wind in Wyoming."

—CARRIE (Won't "get busy" the night before a race because she hates "the leakage.")

"You can't bank your progress. I was running 12-mile-long runs in preparation for a half-marathon, then I broke my toe. Couldn't run for six weeks. Start all over. Every time. Sucks sometimes."

—BERTINA (When she had surgery on her heel—another break from running— she bought herself a "love2run" necklace she still wears every day.)

"I hate the way the back-of-the-pack runners are treated at bigger races. It's never anything overt, but it's hard not to feel 'different' when you cross the finish line, and all the food is gone, the crowds have dwindled, and sometimes there are no medals left."

—KIMBERLY (PS: "The difference between my first marathon (six-hour finish) and my second (five hours) was shocking. All finishers should get the same joyous experience, regardless of speed.")

"That I'm not better at it."

—SARA (Wants to run a major marathon: Chicago, New York, or, ideally, Boston. "I'd be fundraising for that baby!")

EXPECTATIONS ARE EVERYTHING:
A TALE OF THREE HALF-MARATHONS
by Alisa Bonsignore

ACT I: THE BIG BREAK

I'm not exactly what you'd consider an athlete: I got childhood participation medals for softball and graced the bench of my high school basketball team, entering the game only when we were facing massive deficits in the final two minutes of the game.

But for reasons that still remain unclear, I turned to my husband during the haze of labor and said, "If I live through this, I'm running a half-marathon."

The statement was madness. I had no running friends, no lifelong dream of becoming a distance runner, just some corner of my brain that thought if my body could make it through that kind of pain, anything was possible. True to my word, I lumbered through two half-marathons during the first two years of my son's life.

The first race was the Nike Women's Half, my first race of any length. I was so clueless about running I had no idea training plans existed. I didn't have the good sense to search for one online. I don't think my training ever topped 7 miles–and it was mostly walking, to be honest, with the longest "runs" in the two weeks prior to the race. (Taper? What's a taper?) I did the race in head-to-toe cotton, no fuel (what's GU?), finishing in 2:58 with my North Face jacket tied around my waist because I had no idea bag drops existed.

I wanted to try again the following year, so I signed up for the Philadelphia Half. I looked a bit more like a runner in terms of attire, but still didn't know much more about running than I had the year before. The sum total of my athletic development came from picking up a copy of *Runner's World* at the airport before my flight. Jet-lagged and with barely more preparation than the year prior, I walked most of the "flat, fast course" for an improvement of only two minutes over hilly Nike. I was later humbled to realize that a Philly-area colleague had run the entire race, driven to her home in the distant suburbs, and showered before I even crossed the finish line.

So when a local friend lost her husband to lymphoma, a struggle she eloquently documented on her blog, I saw both a chance to honor his memory and find a little personal redemption by joining Team in Training. This was a huge leap of faith for me. Being awkward and nonathletic for my first thirty-seven years, I had terrible fears about joining any group where my progress—or lack thereof—could be measured. It brought back flashbacks of those basketball games where I knew the only workout I would get would come from the mandatory warm-up where I would miss half my uncontested lay-ups.

My fear turned to petrification when I saw Coach Tim, an Ironman and ultramarathoner with to-die-for calf muscles. *This guy is going to kill me*, I thought. *No way I can keep up with him!* By the end of the five-month season, I realized he was the best kind of coach: one who pushes you to your limits, not his. Not only did Coach Tim teach me how to be a proper runner—talking strength training, speed drills, long runs, and *fartleks*—he taught me to appreciate running by telling me to stop comparing myself to others in the group, and instead focus on tackling the hard stuff like speed and hills. (And I realized when he gets compliments on his calves, which happens often, he just gets flustered. Endearing.)

It took a few weeks to find my zone. I began by starting too fast and trying to pace myself with runners in the front of the pack. With Tim's guidance, I eventually found my groove: running slow but steady in the back of the pack. And that was okay, because I'd never felt so strong, so capable, so . . . athletic. On our last long run before the taper, a course preview in San Francisco three weeks before the race, I wasn't even terribly bothered when I took a wrong turn and extended my ten-miler into nearly fourteen.

That night, still on my "I can do anything" high, I broke my foot. Just rolled it while walking across the kitchen. My ankles were so strong (go ankles!) that my ligaments held tight, but my fifth metatarsal gave way. I heard the pop. Just the tiniest little pop, followed by me muttering panicked obscenities. The this-can't-be-happening adrenaline kicked in as I pretended I hadn't heard a thing. When my husband returned from putting our son to bed, I gave a weak, "Ha ha, I think I just broke my right foot," to which he more or less blew me off, because I'd never broken a bone before, and really, what were the odds? I decided to take two ibuprofen and try to sleep it off.

By morning, there was no mistaking the injury. I hopped into urgent care and hobbled out with a giant, black immobilizer boot and a shiny pair of crutches. Not a suitable replacement for the shiny Tiffany bauble, Nike's version of a medal, which I was expecting to symbolize my five months of hard work, by the way.

I'd gone from running 13.8 miles in a training run to hopping thirteen feet from kitchen to couch, depressed and demoralized. I didn't run Nike that October. In fact, I barely did more than limp for the rest of the calendar year.

ACT II: TO PR OR NOT TO PR

"I will never . . . ever . . . stop running again," I wheezed as I struggled through my first "long" Saturday run of the season, a measly 3-mile jaunt along the San Francisco Bay.

Yeah, I'd had plenty of time to get back in shape after ditching the crutches and cane, but life and work had this really irritating habit of getting in the way of my best intentions. My half-assery at the gym didn't exactly prepare me for Coach Tim's strength and endurance sessions, a special pre-training program on Tuesday nights. Track workouts are hard enough without adding in mountain climbers, planks, burpees . . . does anyone know how much I hate burpees?

But before long, I was rolling again, my wheezing laments replaced by long conversations with teammates about everything from the importance of the foam roller to how to streamline fund-raising. As much as I tried to pretend everything was back to normal with my foot, it would ache if my form started to deteriorate. The good news is I wore a minimalist shoe, which meant there was no cushion to hide the discomfort, and I could correct my stride immediately. I adopted a Galloway run/walk program; regular walk breaks of 15 to 30 seconds did wonders to reset my form and keep the aches away, even as the miles added up.

Over twenty weeks and more than 250 training miles, I had come back stronger than ever. Based on our long runs and time calculations, I was on pace to shave close to 30 minutes off my PR. I was ready to take Nike by storm. I talked it over with Coach Tim, and my plan was to do what I'd done in my long runs: slow and steady, contain the exuberance, and stick with the run/walk ratios right from the start. I knew the course well. Plus, Tim's endless hill training had prepared me to slay the toughest spots. I carbo-loaded at the Team in Training dinner the night before, and drifted into an excited sleep while watching hotel HBO. This was my year. I felt unstoppable!

Except that the race was a fiasco from start to finish.

In the starting area surrounding Union Square, it was a total cluster: The porta-potties and bag-check buses were literally within steps of each other. Wall-to-wall women. On the way to meet with my teammates in the proper corral, I got wedged into the wrong corral in a crowd so dense I literally couldn't lift my arm to see if my GPS had found its satellites. Fortunately, I'm 6' 1" and could see over the crowd, but a much shorter woman to my left was having a panic attack from claustrophobia; we all empathized but we couldn't move at all to set her free.

When the race finally began, it was insanity. The seven-minute-milers bobbed and weaved around walkers strolling five abreast. Some runners were on their phones, calling loved ones to let them know they had finally crossed the starting line. I ducked in and out of the thick crowds, up and down curbs trying to dodge obstacles and find a clear path, thinking if I could break through,

I'd be set. Except there was no clear path to be found; all I managed to do was exhaust myself and I was resigned to just walking in the wall-to-wall traffic as the minutes ticked away.

The crowds never thinned. A runner friend, who had raced plenty of times on the San Francisco streets, met me with water and GU at mile 8, near his home. Because I was so far behind my predicted pace, he was certain he had missed me. He marveled at how he had never seen so many people packed so tightly together so deep into a race.

On the bright side, all that walking gave me the chance to appreciate the gorgeous weather. In addition to the hills, San Francisco is also notorious for its fog, so the sunshine and blue skies we had on race day were as rare as a four-leaf clover. We were treated to unobstructed views of the Golden Gate Bridge as we ran along the waterfront, a vantage that usually reveals just a peek of a tower surrounded by a blanket of white.

Still, by the time I passed Coach Tim in Golden Gate Park near mile 11, I tried to avoid eye contact in the hope he wouldn't see me. I'm sure he could see the steam blowing out my ears. I was nowhere near my goal time of 2:30 and perilously close to finishing even slower than my PR. He offered a few words of encouragement, but there really wasn't anything to say. I wasn't his first runner he saw, and we all struggled with feeling out of control. I crossed the finish line at 2:46, waited ninety minutes for a bus back to Union Square, and vowed I would never run this race again.

Maybe I wouldn't even run again.

ACT III: THE SLOW START

It was spring when I got the call from the Team in Training offices asking if I would be a captain for the season, which meant I'd be taking on the same half-marathon for a third time. My brain screamed "no! No! NO!" but my ears heard my mouth say, "Yes." My husband stared at me in disbelief, convinced I'd lost my mind.

Four weeks later, we hit a three-miler through Emeryville on a gorgeous May morning, the first run of the season. I was surprised by how much my winter of Zumba classes had done for maintaining my fitness, but it was obvious my left IT band was being a real bitch. *No matter*, I thought; I'd just go home and roll it out. I had plenty of practice doing that.

It was no better at Tuesday track practice or the following Saturday's run, but it wasn't until I went for a Monday morning hike that I knew something was seriously wrong. I limped back to my car and fought back tears on the drive home. When I tried the foam roller, I couldn't even touch any spot between my left hip and knee without searing pain. I employed the same tactic I had with my foot: ignoring it for as long as possible. Shockingly, that strategy wasn't any more successful this time around. Within a few days, even walking had become an issue.

My physical therapist did some preliminary tests to make sure I hadn't done anything serious. Then he had me roll on to my stomach and raise my leg against his pressure. "Press against my hand," he said. I couldn't. There was no resistance at all. "Wow," he said. "You have a really weak glute on this side."

We traced my weak ass back to my broken foot. Because my quads had been overcompensating, carrying the work of muscles I didn't use during my eight weeks of immobilization, I'd created a serious kink in my IT band. I went to his office twice a week as he used his evil Graston Technique instrument to break up my IT band adhesions. I was in so much agony after those sessions that I got an extra upper-body workout by pulling myself up the banister to the rehab room for the week's prescribed exercises.

At that point, I wasn't entirely sure I'd be able to go back to running. I was struggling even to walk, and it became clear the PT exercises were not optional.

As my team increased its mileage, I became obsessed with getting better, doing my squats and lunges twice a day at home, using my TRX to keep me and my weak ass from toppling over.

Each Tuesday I cheered my teammates at track practice, feeling nearly as demoralized and broken as I had when I was on crutches. Each Saturday I watched my teammates tackle the long runs. I stood alone in the parking lot, squatting and lunging as park maintenance workers watched, no doubt wondering what I was doing. There's nothing quite so humbling as feeling your body is incompetent, especially when you don't know if the situation is temporary or long-term.

I spent nearly eight weeks watching, talking, and enduring Graston. By the time I was cleared to run again in early August, I was way behind. This time, I found myself lumbering along, hanging in the back of the pack. I knew I was moving slower than ever before, so I stopped my usual flow of data: no GPS, no Runkeeper, and absolutely no tracking of progress other than how I felt at the end of the run. My times were irrelevant; I just felt lucky to be out there.

As race day drew near, I set no goals. My plan was to start in the back to pace and encourage my teammates, many of whom were worried about just getting through and finishing ahead of the SAG wagon. That was my entire plan. No times, no PRs, and no goals other than to give others a boost when needed.

Race day dawned, and the Nike organizers had dramatically improved the starting corrals and bag drop, making for a relaxing and enjoyable prerace experience. Runners were dancing, stretching (yes, there was room for that!), and waving to the residents of the apartments above us, who were watching in their pajamas with their coffee. Everyone I knew was able to start in her proper corral with no fuss, fight, or crowds to dodge.

I ran my intervals right from the start. I listened—truly listened—to the bands and the incredible gospel choir stationed along the Embarcadero. I encouraged teammates and complete strangers, offering gels and pacing assistance for those who were struggling to keep going. I high-fived little kids on the sidewalks. I chatted with strangers about everything from their cool gear to interesting city landmarks. I stopped and played on-course photographer for complete strangers who wanted to document their races. Because the race was more organized and the crowds were thinner, I could follow my Galloway program, running and walking at the proper intervals without my pace being dictated by everyone around me. It was relaxed and effortless.

By the time I ran into Coach Tim at the same spot as the previous year in Golden Gate Park, I was beaming. I shouted his name and we trotted along together, chatting. He punched me in the arm and made fun of the fact I was in such a good mood. I laughed, and he sent me on my way to catch up with a teammate to give her the extra push to meet her goal time. I was beaming in my finish-line photo.

My official time? It was 2:52, within 6 minutes of my PR. It was a surprisingly perfect way to close the curtain on my third, and likely final, act with Nike. Geographical proximity to home aside, who in her right mind willingly runs the hills of San Francisco for three consecutive years?

Maybe now I need to give that "fast and flat" Philly course another shot.

TAKE IT *From* A MOTHER
A FAIRY RUNMOTHER MATERIALIZES AND GIVES YOU $200 TO SPEND ON SOMETHING RUNNING-RELATED. WHAT DO YOU SPEND IT ON?

"Probably cute running tops. I can talk myself into spending money on shoes, bras, entry fees, and pants as 'necessary,' but tops feel extravagant."

—MEGAN (Did the two-day Avon Breast Cancer Walk in honor of her sister-in-law two years in a row before she got bored with walking and started to run.)

"A housekeeper or cook so I have more time to run."

—RANDI (Once she could run 30 minutes on the treadmill without stopping, she started to run outside.)

"No question: massage or extra chiropractor visits!"

—ALISON (Has heard SBS talk about emptying the [energy] tank during a race, "but I'm kind of afraid to go all the way there.")

"Race entry to the Nike Women's Marathon—the half—and a new top. Have to look cute in the pictures, right?"

—KATIE (When on a training plan, she'll "move mountains to get a run done. When I'm not, eh, I'll go later.")

"Pedicures and beverages for my running friends in the middle of a training cycle. That's running related, right?"

—JOANN (When her pal offered her ChapStick during the Twin Cities Marathon, she replied, "I'm good. I still have all this Vaseline in my pits." When a guy near them said, "That's TMI." She thought, "Dude, you don't know a thing about TMI.")

"A nice hotel room to stay in before a big race."

—ALESIA (Walks at every mile mark during a run. "That's when I drink or grab a gel.")

"On an airline ticket to Long Beach so I can run along my beloved beach path."

—JANET (Her dream race: "Any race in which my husband and I race all out and I win!")

"New shoes, ChapStick, Nuun, and a Badass Mother Runner tank top!"

—MELISSA (Treat after a long run: margarita and Dove chocolates. "Love reading the notes inside the wrappers.")

"Babysitting. I would love not to have to run in the middle of the night or the butt crack of morning."

—CHANDRA (Has five kids, ages nine to one, plus spent the last two years fostering children with, "serious baggage. I started running because I had to do something to find sanity. Alcohol only helps so much.")

"Cute running clothes. I look much more stylish in my running life than I do in my regular life."

—TERRY (Almost always has to end her run on an even number. "My mileage-logging OCD self doesn't handle decimals very well.")

"A coach. It's time for specific guidance on what I need to do to become a better runner."

—KELLY (Usually feels stronger when she's on the cusp of her period.)

"Really good sports bras. The older I get, the more I realize I need better bras, but they're so expensive."

—CORTNEY (Q: Why did you start running? A: "I don't know. Is that a bad answer?")

"A new brand of shoes just to try them out. I have bought the exact same style of shoe about five times, and I wonder if there is something even better for me out there, but I hate to waste the money if the answer is no."

—JILL (Only loses her motivation to train "when the distance of the looming race freaks me out.")

"One word: Athleta!"

—NANCY (Has never had a major running injury in thirty years of running. "Hope I'm not jinxing myself by admitting that here.")

"Oh, that's tough. A day at the spa after a race sounds enticing."

—KRISTIN (Relies on running to ease her depression. "Even my coworkers can tell if I haven't run in a few days.")

DEFYING GRAVITY
by Dimity McDowell

Becky, Katherine, Jean, and I are playing hooky on a Thursday in late June. Between us, we have ten kids, and all of them are out of school. We've asked our husbands to get to work late and set up babysitters so we can head south to Colorado Springs, about an hour's drive from our homes in Denver, and do a training run up a portion of Pikes Peak. In about two months, we're taking on the Pikes Peak Ascent, a half-marathon that climbs the mountain and finishes at 14,050 feet.

Two of my friends are former collegiate athletes, and all have marathon finishing times that start with three. Read: They are too speedy for me to train with on a daily basis. But long runs, especially those involving a drive to the trailhead to hit unfamiliar trails, are so much better—and safer—with friends, even if I'm chasing them the whole way.

I can't tell if it's true nerves or just politically correct posturing, but in the car, there's a lot of talk about not being able to complete the Ascent. These three women are all impressively tough and healthy. Plus, they live in Colorado, so altitude isn't a huge issue. Always a middle child and now a mother, I try to soothe their fears. "We could get to the top today if we wanted to," I tell them. "Honestly, we could all get up there in less than six-and-a-half hours—the race cut-off time—today."

It's the truth, even for slower, hate-to-climb me. My body, while injury prone, is naturally strong. Second-grade teachers used to tell me gently not to hug my friends so tightly. After college, I won a World Championship in rowing—and when I had a small breakdown about my abilities before the regatta, my coach told me I was the main motor in the four-woman boat. Nearly twenty years after my rowing career ended, I still have defined arm muscles—even though I can only do, on a good day, five "real" push-ups in a row. And last year, I nabbed sixteenth place in my age group in my first Ironman triathlon, after speedwalking most of the marathon.

I'm not saying scaling nearly eight thousand feet over 13.4 miles is a gimme. It'll take about as long as a marathon does and send my quads begging for relief. I am saying I know my muscles can do it. My physical body is the constant in my life, my lowest common denominator. Even though my lower back creaks every morning, I know I'll be able to take stairs two at a time; lift and carry big bags of potting soil; and, if I had to, run a half-marathon on an hour's notice. (The running form and finishing time might not be pretty, but I could do it.)

We're now about an hour into the climb, and the fog this morning is both beautiful and eerie. My three pals are significantly farther in front of me, which doesn't bother me. Even though this is the first time for all of us on this trail, there's pretty much only one way up and one way down. But when the trail makes a well-marked left turn into fog so thick I can barely see my feet, I freak out.

"Are you guys up there? Becky? Katherine? Please stop and wait!" I know Jean, the lead jackrabbit, is way too far up to hear me. But they're all wearing headphones, and I get no reply. I pick up the pace, and they stop to regroup. Within ten minutes, I catch up, and after huffing and puffing out my story, we have a laugh and keep moving up.

If my body is a workhorse, my brain is a foal: unexpectedly wobbly at times, prone to bursts of galloping, liable to wander off if there isn't a fence. One minute, I'm bobbing along and feeling loved. Then, without warning, a thick fog appears, and my head goes haywire. I have no perspective, am ridiculously anxious, and feel uncontrollably sad. Sometimes, when I'm in the fog, I want to barter: a slice of my shoulder muscles for some levity in my life; 20 percent of my glute power in exchange for unexpected, genuine smiles; another layer of fat around my abs so I never break down unexpectedly in public again.

The winter I signed up for the Ascent was not the best season of my life. There's no easy way to say this, so I'll just put it out there: I felt suicidal. I'm not sure I really wanted to die, but I sure thought about it a lot. I was done. Over my head that never stopped spinning, sick of never experiencing peace, let alone happiness. The idea of going through forty or so more years of life feeling mentally strung-out and exhausted was so unappealing I rationalized my family would be better off without me.

As I drove to pick up my two kids at elementary school, I fantasized about getting in a car accident that would take just my life and not hurt anybody else. Other times, I thought I'd overdose on something, or maybe I'd just buy a gun and end it. Most of the time, though, I pictured a white-walled room with gentle light streaming in and an empty bed with a fluffy white comforter, welcoming me with a folded-down corner. That's how I see heaven—soft and clean and quiet—and that winter, it was the most inviting place I could imagine, even if I had to leave this world to get there.

There was nothing traumatic like a death or a frightening medical diagnosis that sent me into this bleak state of mind, which made it seem worse. I know grief eventually moves on; depression just hovers. And the fact I have a life with only first-world problems made me believe I was a selfish, ungracious fool for feeling so terrible. I have running water and a full fridge, a car that works, and a loving husband who likes to care for the car and genuinely loves to fold our laundry. We have two healthy, smart kids; we are on the way to owning our house in a safe neighborhood; and while our financial status wouldn't make Suze Orman beam, we pay our bills on time and can afford occasional vacations, especially when my generous parents spring for lodging.

Yet in this lowest of lows, packing lunches, wrangling teeth brushing, answering e-mails, and other daily tasks seemed as daunting as a 10 x 800-meter workout at the track. As I trudged through the day, I found myself living in a whole new stratosphere of sadness. In the grocery store, I passed by the recycling bins for plastic bags, saw piles of plastic bags, bulging with many more empty, plastic bags, and wept over global warming and the environment. (This is after the photoshopped cover models on women's magazines in the checkout line made me despondent.)

I'd wake up in the middle of the night and dwell on the fact my sisters and I never just pick up the phone to check in. To quiet my mind, I'd turn on NPR at 3:14 a.m. to hear the BBC report about potential genocide in the Central African Republic or another humanitarian crisis, which only revved my mind's RPMs. After yet another tossing-and-turning night, I'd head to a Girls on the Run practice, but instead of gabbing with the other volunteer coaches as the girls circled the school on foot—something I usually love—I'd run a bit with a girl, stop on a corner by myself, and cheer them on. This way, I could be by myself and only yell occasional words of encouragement. Otherwise, clapping was sufficient.

On a March afternoon, my seven-year-old son, practicing his multiplication tables at the kitchen counter, asked me, "Mom, why do you cry so much?" Which of course sent me into the bathroom to use about half a box of Kleenex. And at a therapy session, my husband, Grant, said something that broke my heart even more: "For as long as I've loved you, you've never seemed happy."

As you might guess, depression didn't just knock on my door last winter. Both sides of my family have a history rich in sad, anxious thoughts. For most of my twenties, I pretended I could just use my brute strength to get through depression's genetic force; *I am NOT going to let it get me*, I thought, as I walked two and one half miles home from my first job in Manhattan. (This was after I ran the big loop in Central Park and walked the same distance to work.) In hindsight, I was merely exhausting myself, but I learned then how therapeutic forward movement can be.

Grant and I got married when I was twenty-eight. After that, I stopped busying myself with what flavor wedding cake we were going to have, but a whole bunch of firsts—first move together, first dog, first miscarriage, first house purchase, first baby—kept my mind preoccupied during most of my early thirties. I ran through it all, minus the pregnancy; even though I didn't realize it at the time, every run was the low-dose antidepressant I needed to jump-start my day.

When I run, my mind takes a deep, yogic, cleansing breath. The rhythm of my feet creates a mental peace I've been unable to find anywhere else: not in church, meditation, a therapist's office, or Grant's arms. On a run, choosing joy feels as effortless as blitzing down a hill. On a run, my glass isn't half empty; it's as full and refreshing as the water bottle I clutch in my hand. On a run, all those things on Lululemon bags—*dance, sing, floss, travel, be happy*—seem like great ideas, not admonitions of what I am not inclined to do. I rarely feel worry or anguish on a run. I've shed tears on a run, but even when it's been in relation to a death or something similarly traumatic, grateful-ness and love—not depression—brought on the waterworks.

Running, I am the person I want to be when I am standing still.

Problem was, the few, reluctant miles I put in that winter weren't the balancing elixir I have, for two decades, relied on them to be. I completed the aforementioned Ironman the previous June, and seven months later, I still felt hungover from pedaling nowhere on my bike for four-hour rides in the basement, from eighty-minute sessions in the pool during which my fingers shriveled to raisins, from double-digit runs. The miles were predictably positive, but there were just so dang many of them.

That winter, I didn't need to train for another Ironman—or even a 10K—but I rarely put in enough time to get the endorphin rush that courses through my veins after 4 or so miles of running or an hour of steady pedaling on the bike. I need that flood of happiness at least five times a week, and I was hitting it maybe three days, usually two. When I consistently chose my bed over a sweat session in the morning, I also made other downward-spiral choices: grilled cheese and other fog-inducing foods for lunch; handfuls of sugar throughout the day; a generous glass of wine at 4 p.m.; not returning calls or texts from family and friends.

Obviously, too many peanut M&M's and ignored messages from my mom didn't make me suicidal, but they were factors in a perfect storm. Genetics created hurricane-like conditions, and then everything else spiraled into them. I overdid it with Ironman, which made me not want to exercise on, say, a random Tuesday, which made me sleep horribly that night, which convinced me not to get up to run on Wednesday, which sunk me down even further, which made five Oreos at 10 a.m. seem like an acceptable mid-morning snack, which sent me into a sugar high and then flung me down deeper than I was before, which made me disconnect from my support network. Working at home alone through an especially cold and snowy winter also whipped everything into a frenzy, and the cyclone swept me away.

Fortunately, I kept taking my meds—meds, mind you, I'd promised myself I'd only take for a year after I had my second kid, who is now eight. I spent some time in therapy, both with and without Grant. And even though my sleep sucked, I went to bed early. Sometimes before eight. Being prone with my eyes shut was, thankfully, an acceptable alternative to sending myself to that fluffy-white-comforter place I longed for most days.

One day at the library, while my almost eleven-year-old daughter perused the young adult section and my son bemoaned there weren't more Captain Underpants books to read, I saw a book called *The Depression Cure* on a display table. I checked it out, and while a lot of it was stuff I already knew—quality sleep and regular exercise are key to keeping your mood positive—it emphasized, among other things, the importance of a diet rich in omega-3s, daily exposure to light, and social connectedness (not the kind found through a keyboard). I gave it a try, hitting up the Whole Foods vitamin aisle, dragging a chair out to the middle of our lawn to soak up sun while I worked, and reaching out to one friend I knew would make me laugh. I didn't have the courage to tell her how deep in a hole I was.

I pulled out of a local half-Ironman I'd signed up for before I realized how much spark I'd lost, and I tried not to dwell on the fact I gave up on something before I even started, which didn't sit well with my work ethic. Sensing the Ascent was the perfect event, I refocused on getting up the mountain. I had a neighborhood posse to keep me going, and it's not the type of race where I was going to obsess over splits. (How long does it take to climb seven-hundred-fifty boulder-strewn feet over a mile? No freakin' idea.) Still, I had to put in some miles and get on a schedule. Even if my muscular legs could get me to the top on any given day, I wanted a race-day adventure, not a sufferfest.

I don't know when, exactly, my thoughts stopped being subsumed with figuring out a way not to be here anymore. I know all the healing steps I took helped, but I also realize I'm kidding myself if I think I'm done with depression. It's like I was in the middle of a crazy downpour all winter, then slowly, week by week, the rain tapered off. Finally, it was misty one week, and the sun peaked through the clouds the next.

Before the Ascent, I have no nerves or expectations. *Just a great day to climb a big mountain*, I tell myself as I watch my trio of pals go off in the fast wave ahead of me. Thirty minutes later, I'm lining up under a bluebird sky, and we're off. The climbing starts right away; the first mile and a half of the Ascent, while on pavement, isn't easy. My calves strain as my body tries to find a rhythm among the hundreds of runners of various speeds around me. Some are gunning it so they can be in a better position when we hit the narrow Barr Trail that will take us up the mountain; some are conservative, walking as soon as an incline gets significant. I'm somewhere in the middle.

We funnel onto the trail, a single-file line of athletes in bright tops with hydration packs of every stripe. Because of the demanding grade and crowds, there's very little running going on. It's more like fast hiking and, sometimes, slow walking. I can almost feel the panting breath of the person behind me, which makes me claustrophobic and mentally scrambled. Focusing on the rocky, rutted trail requires most of my energy; what's left goes to making sure I don't clip the heels of the person in front of me. When I'm about to plow somebody over, I wait for a wider spot in the trail—not really enough room for two people, but it'll do—and I say, "On your left," power up my quads, and brush by.

My sports watch only displays the time of day; I didn't want any kind of splits or mile markers, so I left my GPS at home. I know we started at 7:30, and my plan is to suck down one vanilla GU— the bland flavor works well for me—every 30 minutes. It's more than I would eat in a regular race, but I don't want to bonk a thousand feet from the summit. Around 9 a.m., we hit an aid station, and sugar-loving me is so excited to see Jelly Bellys, I grab a handful of them as my gel substitute. Without thinking, I shovel most of them in my mouth and immediately regret it: Flavors of cappuccino and cantaloupe and cinnamon mix in my mouth. If I wasn't feeling out of sorts before, I certainly am now.

As I burp up the flavor of toasted marshmallow, I realize I have no idea if I'm working too hard or not hard enough, and I am far from the happy place running transports me to. To ease my anxiety, I distract myself. "Is that where we're going?" I say to nobody in particular as I catch a glimpse of a hard, bald peak that looks so far off it could well be located in Alaska. "Yes," says the woman in front of me. "Just acknowledge that it's there, then do your best to forget about how far away it looks."

She's my kind of girl, I think, and start grilling her with questions. She's a local and has biked up Pikes Peak on the road; hiked up it "countless times"; and has taken the cog railway to the top. "It's about to get a little easier," she says, and she's right. The incline lessens a bit, and the easiest section of the course is upon us.

"Have a great race," I tell her as I speed through an aid station where she lingers. The pack of athletes, formerly a crazy long tapeworm, has now broken into hundreds of sections of inchworms. I still don't have a rhythm, but at least I have some space. When I see longer stretches of runnable terrain in front of me, I let my legs open up as much as my aching back allows. (Nonstop climbing, it turns out, is amazingly easy for your joints. Hard on the back and hip muscles, though.)

I pick the pace up regularly, even if there are only eight steps of running before I hit another inchworm. After doing this maneuver a few times, I realize speeding up to stop requires a lot of energy, whereas maintaining my ambitious hike and slowly reeling in the group ahead is much more efficient—and, more importantly, feels less frantic. Life lessons on the trail.

I finally get above treeline—about 3.3 miles to go—and the trail goes from puzzle pieces of rocks, roots, shade, and sun to just rocks as far as the eye can see. I can hear vuvuzelas, those plastic horns popular at the 2010 World Cup, being blown at the finish line, and my soaked shirt starts to dry from the first breeze I've felt all day. A young woman in small, tight, florescent-green shorts, the kind that flatter only a select few, passes me. Her attitude matches her peppy shorts. "Look around!" she blurts. "How amazing is this?" Despite not exactly knowing where I was, effort-wise, on the previous 10 miles, I'm feeling good. (Much better than the people around me resting on rocks, anyway.) I decide I'm going to do what it takes to stay with her. I want to soak up her enthusiasm and, hey, I wouldn't mind having her buns, either.

I don't glue myself to her, but when she passes somebody, I try to go with her. That works for about a mile. She's on the move, and my glutes in my mom-length black Lycra shorts can't compete. I'm not really bummed about that, though. We've still got more than 2 miles to go, which means at least another 50 minutes of climbing. (I've heard the final few miles take 20 to 30 minutes each.)

Okay, Dimity, I tell myself, *it's up to you to settle in, regroup, and finish this thing.* I stay in the back of the inchworm groups that seem to match my pace, and pass only when someone is clearly struggling and the path is somewhat accommodating. When a young guy whizzes by me, then plops himself on a boulder a few steps later, I prod him along. "No sitting! You've got a great pace." He thanks me, rises, and keeps ascending. A search-and-rescue team standing on massive rocks around the corner of a switchback is quacking out "The Muppet Show" theme and other gems on kazoos, but I can't cheer them on like those around me do. I'm weary and wiped from the relentless uphill.

This should be the place in my story where I say I climbed out of a scary hole, and I've almost climbed to the top of Colorado, and I'm euphoric. That'd be neat, but I'm not. I am, however, definitely grateful to be alive on this Saturday in August, with a text on my phone from my daughter that reads, "You're going to rock it, Mom!"; a throbbing toenail on my left foot; and three friends ahead of me, with whom I will soon share a beer while we recount our races.

As I finally see the finish line I've heard for the past 3 miles, my Jelly Belly overload feels as far away as last winter does. I'm grateful for that, too. I exhale, whisper a soft thanks, and then do what I've always done: I let my legs carry me.

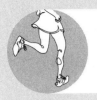

WHAT A MOTHER RUNNER LOOKS LIKE . . .

IN HER TWENTIES

Case Study:

Rae, age twenty-four

Washington, Missouri

Mother to one child: age two

Athletic history: I did gymnastics, and played roller hockey and volleyball up to middle school, and did a little horseback riding. In high school, I played some volleyball. College was a lazy time for me, but I started doing Zumba at the encouragement of my now-BRF (best running friend).

Started running: At age twenty-two. I was definitely ready to lose the baby (and the college) weight.

First run, post-baby: My younger sister runs cross-country and track in high school, and my mom is a runner. I saw how much they love it. I had a natural birth with my son, so I told myself I was tough enough to run at least a mile. Six weeks postpartum, I asked my sister, then sixteen, if she would slow down by 6 minutes a mile so I could run with her. She did. I was wheezing and trying not to vomit, but I didn't die, which is good. I wanted to walk so badly, but I didn't want to let my sister see me quit.

Typical running day: My husband is a state trooper, and he works two weeks of days, then two weeks of nights, so I can't get into any real pattern. I run when he's home; sometimes it's early morning, sometimes it's night. I never run with my son, Maverick. We have a running stroller, but I hate it. I feel constrained when I'm pushing him. And he doesn't like being strapped in. So when we go together, he's mad, and I'm mad, and nothing good comes of that.

Typical running week: I try to get out at least three times, including a long run on the weekend, but the number of miles really varies.

Speed bumps: I have exercise-induced asthma. But I haven't taken a hit off my inhaler in more than a year, and I stopped carrying it six months after I started running. I rarely feel like I'm losing my breath anymore.

Maverick has the immune system of a beast. The few times I've missed running because I needed to stay home to take care of him, I get mad and yell at my husband because I'm frustrated I can't run, then I tell him that's why I'm crabby and things settle down. I get through the day, have some ice cream after dinner, and feel better.

Body concerns: I've heard childbirth does weird things to your body, but I haven't had any problems. I had years of what felt like continual sprained ankles, which resulted in damaged nerves in one of my legs. When I started running, I was nervous I'd hurt my legs more, but it's only made my whole body stronger.

When I was nursing and running, all I wanted was a hundred Moving Comfort Fiona bras. Alas, I only had one, which I washed over and over.

The million-dollar question: We want to have more kids, but I'm currently training for the Twin Cities Marathon, my first, so we're thinking no more babies right now. I have had dreams I'm pregnant and wake up wondering if I should take a test, but so far I'm not. Maverick was a happy fluke—I got pregnant while on birth control—so anything is possible.

Best part of running: The peace. I can shut off my mind and just rock to the music or focus on a book; I love Tina Fey's *Bossypants* and the Harry Potter series. There's no chance of interruption from my little one. I also love the challenge. I win every run.

Finding balance: Family support is really big for me. I can't fathom not having it. I'm training for my first marathon, and I swear, I've apologized a thousand times for my training time. "This is what you want to do," my husband says, and encourages me to go. We realized life is much better with me running.

Perspective motherhood brings to running: When I started running, I thought about giving birth. While in labor, I kept reminding myself there's an end result to this weird, painful, uncomfortable situation. There's a joy waiting for me at the end. I think about running the same way: I could be on a run that's too hot or is uncomfortable because I ate fast food earlier in the day, but when it's done, the joy is always waiting for me.

Plus, even the bad runs eventually end. I come home and get on the floor to do some push-ups, and there's a baby on my back. I can't *not* laugh.

Parting words: Today I woke up at 6 a.m. to run. I just did it, and now I feel great. I wish it was 1 p.m. right now, but it's only 10:30 a.m. I'll make it to naptime.

IN HER THIRTIES

Case Study:

Susan, age thirty-four

Escondido, California

Mother to four kids: ages twelve, nine, six, and three (plus two dogs, two cats, and a variable number of fish)

Athletic history: I figure-skated as a preteen/teenager. I actually skated at the same rink as Tonya Harding in Oregon; she was my idol. I pretty much sucked at any other sport I was forced to do in school. I still can't swim to save my life, or anyone else's. The hubs is trying to make me take an adult swim class this summer, but I'm way too embarrassed.

Started running: I got serious about running at age thirty-two. My sister talked me into trying the Couch to 5K program after my fourth baby. I'm so grateful to her; I'm a much happier, healthier, well-balanced person now.

Typical running day: I don't really have one.

My husband and I are both nurses, so one of us is always home with the kids. I work two twelve-hour shifts weekly, with an hour commute each way, so those are always my off days, although I try to get in a few strength training exercises—lunges, squats, some arm moves with weights—before I head out.

On the days we're both home, I run outside without a stroller, but usually with our dog. She turns every run into a *fartlek* session, sprinting like crazy, then stopping to sniff something or to poop.

When I'm home alone, I either run on the treadmill or with the stroller. Last year, the two-year-old was in the stroller and the five-year-old would ride on a little ledge on the front and jump off and run with me. This year, he's starting kindergarten, so I'm looking forward to having only one kid on the run.

I would love to be an early morning runner, but it's just too hard. The baby wakes up and has a little protest; it just works out for me to go later, after I've dropped the older kids at school.

Typical running week: I run four or five days a week. Each run is from 3 to 13 miles, so I get to about 20 to 25 miles a week. I'm trying to get up to 30 miles weekly and am gearing up for my first marathon, the Carlsbad Marathon, this winter.

Speed bumps: Although my kids are proud of me—when we're driving and see a runner, my five-year-old says, "There's a Badass Mother Runner like you"—they don't always like that I run.

When I put on my shoes, my youngest sits on top of the treadmill and declares, "No running, Mama." I bribe him with candy or the show *Yo Gabba Gabba* or whatever distraction is available. And then there was the time when one of my kids chucked a toy piano at me while I was on the treadmill. I was laughing pretty hard, but I got off. *(Editor's note: During the phone interview for this profile, the youngest heard Susan say "running," and he kept repeating, "No running, Mama.")*

Physical challenges: I've had shin splints and problems with my calves and hip. I just started going to barre class and need to pull out the Sage Rountree *The Athlete's Guide to Yoga* DVD, which is gathering dust on my shelf. I also occasionally do strength training DVDs from *Women's Health*, which make me faster and stronger.

I also have some lower-back pain, but that only flares up after driving my husband's commuter car, not my roomy Suburban. Weird.

Mental challenges: I'm very competitive. I was hoping to slide in under two hours in a recent half-marathon, and I was pretty bummed about not getting it. I'm also a perfectionist. I repeat a whole week of training if I miss one workout. When I can't run, I get stressed about it. I'll jump on the treadmill, even if it's a long run.

Perspective motherhood brings to my running: Being a mommy to my four amazing children has been the greatest blessing of my life. I want to be around for them for a long, long time, and running will help me get there. Also, I know if I can survive forty-eight continuous hours of labor (thanks, child number one!), I can survive four hours of running, one step at a time.

Parting words: I have the Mirena IUD, so I get zero periods. Awesome! Wait, I take that back; since the youngest baby is now weaned, Aunt Flo has returned. Bummer.

IN HER FORTIES

Case Study:

Jennifer, age forty-four

Raleigh, North Carolina

Mother to two kids: ages fourteen and twelve

Athletic history: I was a competitive swimmer through my childhood and high school. Outside of hoisting twelve-ounce curls of cheap beer in college, I was sedentary. Feeling plump in my mid-twenties, I started aerobics, walking, and dabbling in running.

Started running: More than 2 miles at a time? At age thirty-eight. Six years later, I've done sixteen marathons and three ultramarathons (anything longer than 26.2 miles).

Typical running day: I get up at 5:25 a.m. to get to CrossFit at 6, which I do three times a week. Head home, get the kids ready for school, then head to the office. I used to be a morning runner, usually by myself with one of my dogs, but now I've got two younger coworkers who have kindly been referred to by friends as my "run pups." (They are twelve and twenty-three years younger than I am.) They're training for their first marathon, so we train together. One of the pups lives in my neighborhood, so we run in the morning, but if we miss that because of oversleeping or a morning meeting, we run at lunch or after work.

Typical running week: I run four times a week and do CrossFit three times a week. Like running, CrossFit pushes me out of my comfort zone. I am faster, as well as physically and mentally stronger, and I finish races feeling the best I ever have. One day a week I have a double workout of running in the morning and CrossFit in the evening.

Speed bumps: Is it awful to say I currently have none? I started running when my husband began struggling with alcohol addiction. I learned early on I couldn't control the addiction, but I could control my response, and I turned to running to stay sane. Running helped me put things in perspective, do something for myself, and be strong for my family. My husband is completely supportive of my running; he understood running was my healing and that he and I were working together to overcome our obstacles. While I am thankful for every mile and my BRFs—best running friends—I am most proud of my husband's continued fight and his celebration of sobriety (five years and counting).

Physical challenges: I've only been sidelined briefly with minor running injuries, so I feel pretty lucky in that respect. I occasionally have night sweats, but I don't think I'm hitting perimenopause yet. I actually recently confirmed with my OB I have no signs of menopause yet. Yeah! I don't feel like I'm in my mid-forties; most days, I feel just as young as my twenty-something friends.

Mental challenges: Not getting caught up in the competitive side of running: I run to complete, not compete. I am working on accepting that running is my serenity, on being okay that I am not always gunning for a personal record or Boston qualifier. Focusing on others or the clock steals my enjoyment, and it's too much work. I just want to continue to run injury-free and happy.

Like mother, not like kids: My son is a hockey player, and my daughter is a competitive swimmer. I wish they were doing 5Ks with me, but they haven't taken an interest in running. Yet. When I was growing up, my mom was really into aerobics, and it was so embarrassing for me that she did it wearing leotards, leg warmers, headbands . . . the full package. I wouldn't do aerobics because my mom did it. Maybe my daughter won't do it because of me, but I'll happily wait and see.

Perspective motherhood brings to my running: For me, running is both personal and social. It is both time for me to be alone in my head, and it is also often the only social outlet I get outside of work and family. Whether I'm running alone or with my pups, the time and endorphins make me be a better mother and wife. Yes, I am away from my kids, but I am showing them that with a lot of hard work, you can accomplish your goals. It's not always easy. There will be failures and bumps along the way; you just have to try harder the next time. My running is real-life lessons in action.

Parting words: If I died tomorrow, I am positive my eulogy would be centered on my love for endorphins.

IN HER FIFTIES

Case Study:

Nicki, age fifty-three

Endicott, New York

Mother to six kids: ages thirty, twenty-seven, twenty-seven, twenty-six, twenty-four, and twenty

Athletic history: I grew up in the 1960s and early '70s, and there weren't kids' teams sports like there are now. I did things like ride my bike around the neighborhood, but didn't participate in any organized sports in high school and college. I biked through my first pregnancy, but with my second pregnancy—twins—I was placed on bed rest at twenty-six weeks.

Once I had three kids, there was suddenly no time. I was working full time and dealing with three children two and under. I found myself pregnant again and eventually gave up full-time work. I had a friend who was a Jazzercise instructor, and as soon as I had baby four, I started going to her class because they had daycare. For three years in the late 1980s, I Jazzercised at least twice a week. Two more kids followed—at one point I had four kids under five—and it took me until the youngest was twelve to drop the last of the baby weight. It would've been nice to do that earlier in my life.

Started running: A few days shy of my forty-sixth birthday. I needed to outrun my heredity. Both my parents were/are diabetics with high blood pressure, and I realized those diseases were coming for me if I didn't get my act together.

Typical running day: I get up between 5 and 6 a.m. and start working; I'm a freelance writer and like to get some work done before I run. I'll generally run midday, shower, then work some more. But on long-run days, I'll run in the morning; I also join social runs at night sometimes.

Typical running week: I run four or five days a week; running six days is too tough on my body. I generally log between 25 and 35 miles when I'm not on a training schedule. But I'm almost always training for something.

Speed bumps: My biggest hurdle these days is integrating cross-training into my routine. I was at my most fit when I swam three times a week, took a weekly kickboxing class, and was running. But the kickboxing class ended, and the pool hours became too early for me.

Physical challenges: I had a horrible case of plantar fasciitis for an entire summer, and I had to take three months off. I had hoped to run an October marathon that year, but couldn't. That's been my only injury, and after I got over it, I decided I was only going to run half-marathons from here on out to avoid injury. Yet I am running the Marine Corps Marathon this fall. Don't ask me how *that* happened.

One of my biggest concerns is menopause. I wonder how it'll affect my running, and I don't have many friends in a similar situation who I can ask about it. I haven't even had an occasional hot flash yet; I'm as regular as I was when I was twenty. It drives me crazy, but I can't convince my doctor she should just haul away my uterus for no reason.

Running to the rescue: I knew running was mitigating my potential genetic medical issues, but I didn't realize how much it helps me keep everything in control. Recently, I had to fly at the last minute to California to help my ailing mother, and I had to pack, tell my kids, and deal with a guy who wanted to be important in my life. (I'm recently divorced, but had been separated for sixteen years.) I didn't run for a week, and my blood pressure was sky high. (I checked it at the store with my stepfather.) I went for a 3-mile walk that night, and a run the next morning, and the next time I checked it, it was back to normal.

Like mother, not like kids: At first, my kids thought I was crazy to take up running. My oldest has since run some 5Ks—mostly because he was under the influence of a girlfriend. My daughter ran a half-marathon last year. She liked it, but says she has no desire to do it again. She ran a 2:04, and I'm like, "Really? You're done with running?"

Perspective motherhood brings to my running: I have watched two parents battle with debilitating disease, with my mom now fighting what will likely be her last round. She has been one of my biggest supporters through all kinds of turmoil in my life and has encouraged me to run while taking care of her. Hopefully, I'm setting an example my children will follow. There are so many ways to deal with life and stress, and running is the one I have chosen. At least my kids realize there are nondestructive ways to deal with the ups and down of life; running has helped me set that example.

Parting words: I have been a single parent since 1997, and I do not know how parents, single or not, run with younger kids. I am in complete awe of younger mothers who find the time—and drive— to run.

IN HER SIXTIES

Case Study:

Ann, age sixty-five

University City, Missouri

Mother to two kids: ages thirty-eight and thirty-four. One granddaughter: age eight

Athletic history: I was a tomboy as a child, competing with brothers and other boys in the neighborhood. I was also an avid swimmer throughout childhood, and a lifeguard and swim instructor during high school.

Started running: At age twenty-eight I had a new baby, had just moved to Rochester, New York, and wanted to get out and be active. I read a friend's copy of *Runner's World* and a book called *Running for Health and Beauty,* bought a pair of Nike waffle trainers, and just went out and ran for 15 to 20 minutes, then turned around and ran home. No women I knew were really running in 1978—they were into Jane Fonda—and when I talked about it, they looked at me like I had a third eye.

I started running during the time of the Jonestown massacre, and the news reports were devastating. After a run, I'd have a cup of chamomile tea, watch the news, and question humanity's cruelty. To this day, I can't drink chamomile tea.

Typical running day: Even though I keep trying to run in the morning, I just can't. I'm a night person, so I run in the evening, after sunset, when folks are out walking their dogs for the last time before turning in. It's something I look forward to all day and is a nice wind-down. I have lots of reflective gear, flashing lights, and an SOS button on my watch that will alert my husband and daughter with a "Help!" text and GPS for exact location.

Typical running week: I run every other day for 3 to 5 miles in our neighborhood, with long runs of 6 to 10 miles on the weekend. I ramp it up for spring and fall half-marathons, but still run every other day.

Speed bumps: I try to stay away from the "getting old" conversations. I have some non-runner friends who seem to focus on aches, pains, medications. I just don't like that mentality at all.

My times got slower in my forties and fifties; my PR for the half-marathon for my sixties is 2:45, which is 56 minutes slower than my all-time PR I clocked in my early thirties. I focus on having a PR for each decade. I'd like to break 2:40 in the half. I know what I'm physically capable of, and what it takes to get faster. Staying injury-free is always my number one priority.

Physical challenges: I've had just about every running injury possible, and starting over gets harder each time. Coming back after a broken foot, which happened during a racquetball game, was the worst. I don't cope well with injuries, but patience, mindful meditation, and yoga help.

When I went through menopause during my early fifties, running minimized its effects. I definitely didn't want to feel hot flashes when it was eighty degrees out during mile 5 and, thankfully, I didn't get them.

I still need to keep strengthening my core. My legs and quads are strong, but the rest of my body fatigues quickly and my form can be compromised. I don't like running with my shoulders at my ears.

Mental challenges: I don't have many. I've always been a solo, intrinsic runner. I don't care about the medals or awards. Plus, when I'm running, I feel like I'm thirty-five, even though I'm not. Sure enough, though, I typically win age group awards because there are so few women my age running and racing.

Mother Nature runner: I love being in nature in every possible condition—rain, snow, cold, sun—and seeing the minute seasonal changes. For example, two days ago, the lilac wasn't in bloom, and today it is; I smelled it before I saw it. Then there's the overwhelming beauty in the spring with forsythia, dogwood, and Bradford pears blossoming; seeing the same heron in the same pond all summer; acorns and leaves of different sizes and colors on the street; spotting a turtle or fox on the path; the absolute stillness of running at night in the snow and hearing a big plop of snow fall from a tree.

Perspective motherhood brings to my running: My daughters always knew me as a runner, and they cheered me on at races for years. They joined me when they got older, and many of my best running moments include running races, from 5Ks to half-marathons, with my daughters, and run/walking fun runs and 5Ks with my granddaughter.

Parting words: On November 18, 2014, I celebrated my thirty-sixth running birthday and recommitted, as I always do, to the sport. There's no reason not to keep running.

03

SUPPORT:
You Can't Go It Alone

"My faster, way-more-experienced running
friend gradually and patiently got me to
run 5 miles on a trail, which I'd never done
before. I will love her forever for those
Wednesday mornings. And I will always be
willing to run with somebody slower than
I am because of the grace she showed me."

—SARAH

FRIENDS WITH BENEFITS
by Tish Hamilton

Tap, tap, tap, on my left shoulder.

I turned, and there was my friend, her smile big in the bright sunshine, her hair stiff with sweat, her face rimed with salt—as I'm sure mine was, too. We were coming up on mile 23 of the Boston Marathon; who knows how long she'd been chasing me down. The journey to this point had begun, depending on how you looked at it, either three-plus hours or three-plus years ago. I was both delighted to see her and, truth be told, a little dismayed.

"Hi, friend," she said.

If you've ever had a running buddy, you know how valuable she is. You don't ignore the alarm clock when you know she's meeting you on a dark and cold morning; the last miles of a long run aren't so painful when you're gossiping about your neighbors. But the talk isn't always Botox and minivans. On a run, it's easier to share embarrassing secrets and parse painful subjects because you're not looking directly into someone's eyes. Run with a good friend for many miles and eventually you'll reveal something you've never told anyone, with the understanding your secret is safe. What's said on the run stays on the run.

When you do any one activity for long enough—knit, golf, play the ukulele—you find a network of like-minded people. I've been running for twenty-five years, so at this point, I know a lot of runners. (In fact, at this point, I have very few friends who *don't* run.) That said, a truly good running friend is hard to find. Which is what makes them so special. As with any successful relationship, much has to be compatible, starting with how far and how fast you both can run and, critical for all for mothers, the time of day at which you both can get out. And, of course, the elusive factor in the equation: You have to simply like each other, especially when you're meeting in the dark before coffee and spending up to three hours together on weekend long runs. The stars have to align.

I was surprised to see, in a recent Running USA survey of fourteen thousand women, that 42 percent prefer to run alone. I mean, I do have at least one girlfriend—a dear former colleague—who can't stand running with company. Before she had kids, she would run alone from Harlem to Battery Park City on Saturdays and Sundays. Two to three hours, on both days, by herself! And not to train, but just because she enjoyed it. I pressured her into signing up for one marathon. "You run so much! You might as well!" She hated the experience and has never raced again.

Still, when I read that survey, I thought, *Nah, most women don't* prefer *to run* alone, *they just do it because it's easier.* In her book *Maxed Out: American Moms on the Brink,* Katrina Alcorn says one of the first things women lose when they get married and have kids—especially if they're working outside the home—is female friendships. Because (sadly) who has time?

I spend enough time alone with my demons; I don't need to go for a run with them. So I say yes to anyone who asks—as long as I think I can keep up without embarrassing myself. But it doesn't always work out. A running-club acquaintance, whose personal and professional background mirrored mine, always ran just a step or two in front, and talked over her shoulder. Every time I pulled even, she'd pull ahead. Annoying. A few house-moves ago, I had high hopes for another woman who lived a mile away in my suburb; she was roughly my age, my pace, my profession. We could meet by running toward each other before work! And we did for a while, but the truth was—God forgive me—she had one of those nasal, raised-in-Joisey accents and complained a lot. Oh my gawd, it's sew hawt. No, thank you.

Tap, tap, tap. This relatively new running buddy greeting me at mile 23 of the Boston Marathon was a good one, a keeper. Willing, gracious, smart, funny: All the things you treasure in a friend and hope to give back to her. You'd think I'd be overjoyed to see the person who'd paced me through nearly every step of the way of the past three difficult years. So why did I feel my heart sink, just a little?

"I'm not happy," my husband of twenty-plus years had told me one winter morning three years earlier. He wanted out, and my panicky mind went into hyper-overdrive: What would we do about our big, beautiful house? How would we tell our six-year-old daughter? How would I keep up my running as a single parent? I was supposed to start a marathon-training plan the very next day!

When your life unspools, who do you call? My oldest, dearest friend (a runner, of course, but not the one in Boston) was away. She was on a momentous trip to Hawaii to complete her quest to run a marathon in all fifty states. I couldn't wrap my head around the time difference and whether she was running at that very minute, so I texted instead of calling. "Congratulations on your fiftieth state!" I typed and waited about two seconds, my hands shaking, before typing again. "I'm getting divorced." (Imagine receiving that text. I'm still apologizing.)

Every divorcee will tell you how important friends are during the dissolution of a marriage. You lose a lot when you lose a partner, including the person with whom you've navigated every situation, big and small, at a time when you most need someone to help you steer your course. Move closer to work, or stay in the current school district? Buy the house with the attached garage and 1970s cabin kitchen, or the newer kitchen but falling-down shed-garage? Queen bed or full? Yellow bedspread or gray? Decisions became paralyzing. Forward motion kept me going.

Fortunately, after twenty-five years of hitting the road with anyone who'd agree, I had a good collection of friends to join me on healing runs. My friend who truly prefers to run solo came out with me in a torrential downpour during her beach vacation. "Was that thunder?" On one long run with an ultrarunning friend, as we climbed a very steep hill, she said, "I wish there was something I could do to help." To which I replied, "You're doing it right now!" A triathlete friend invited my daughter for a playdate so I could sneak in a six-miler. On a Sunday morning rail-to-trail run, while her husband minded our kids, my social-worker friend let me complain about a therapist who'd advised me to keep my problems in perspective. "Think of all the people in India who don't have indoor plumbing," the therapist had said, which particularly irked me given that the toilet in my new little house clogged so frequently I had to snake it after nearly every poop.

During this maelstrom, I found myself folded into a pint-size chair in a conference with my daughter's first-grade teacher. I had just told her about my family situation, and I was trying not to cry. She took pity on me and changed the subject, saying, "You run marathons, right? There's a teacher on the first-grade team who runs marathons, too. You should get together!"

The divide between a recreational runner for whom breaking four hours in a marathon is a major accomplishment and a professional runner who knocks out a seventeen-miler at 6:20 per mile can seem vast and unconquerable. (Indeed, I could not keep up a 6:20 pace for even a quarter of a mile.) But I have found women all up and down the pace scale appreciate—and even crave—their running friendships. (Does the same hold true for men? I don't know. I don't care about them right now.)

A couple of years ago, Kara Goucher and Shalane Flanagan, two top professional American runners, joined forces to train for the Boston Marathon, and the running world was astonished, baffled, disbelieving. How could two extremely competitive women at the top of their games spend so much time together, sharing a coach and a vision, logging long miles, punishing each other in track sessions, crunching side by side in the gym, then go to the starting line of the marathon and try to beat each other in the same race? After all, only one could win.

Actually, when I say "the running world" was astonished, baffled, disbelieving, I really mean "my boss." He wanted me to interview Kara and Shalane to dissect their training friendship. While I was thrilled to comply, I wasn't the least bit mystified. I mean, why would they *not* want to train together? How great it must've been for each of them to find someone with the same goals, desires, drive, speed. Not to be simple-minded, but they'd have someone to talk to! Someone who got it. And that's exactly what they told me.

"We go out for a run, and we talk and talk and talk," Kara said, three months before their goal marathon. "People will go, 'What do you guys talk about?' And I'm like, 'Everything and nothing.' We've had really deep conversations where we've talked about our childhoods, and then we have other conversations where we talk about the TV we watched the night before."

"There's only one day a week that we don't see each other," said Shalane. "It's amazing we don't run out of things to talk about."

After Ex and I sold the big house, I moved with my daughter into a small house in town ("as is" garage, full bed, yellow-*and*-gray bedspread), which, as it happens, was about half a mile from the first-grade teacher who also ran marathons. "We should run together some time!" we said when we saw each other in the school hallway or at the grocery store, until one of us—probably desperate me—finally said, "Okay, how about Saturday morning?"

The first few runs with a new buddy can be as awkward as a first date. You have to find your pace, your route, your rhythm. And quite frankly, I was intimidated. She was a popular teacher, after all, which is like being a local celebrity, with all the respect and scrutiny that position commands. Tall and thin, with piercing blue eyes. "Stunning," in the words of another mother. Thanks to race results on the Internet, I knew she was younger and faster than me. Not Kara Goucher fast, but fast enough to wake me up.

At first I was vulnerable, cautious, and tentative, and said very little about the divorce. Honestly, it was a relief not to have a shared past that had to be dissected and revised. Unlike my other running friends, she and her husband hadn't known Ex, so we didn't have to worry about divided loyalties or feel rueful about not having him around anymore. A brand-new friendship allowed me to start the difficult task of shaping an identity independent of the past, a process made more endurable with the tonic of a run.

Soon enough Fast Teacher Friend—my nickname for her, to which she objects—and I settled into a routine of running once a week, at 5:30, before school, on the morning my daughter was at her dad's house. Then we started adding miles to a Saturday long run. Then we put a marathon on the calendar and trained together, gradually building up the miles, the conversations, the confidence.

Three years later, we meet up whenever our schedules mesh. We have a Friday loop, a Sunday loop. We leave our houses at an agreed-upon time and meet in the middle. And I can tell you there is no happier sight on a dark, ten-degree morning at 5:30 than a smiling runner coming toward you, arms outstretched for a greeting hug—remember, she's a teacher. "I'm so glad to see you!" We notice each other's new shoes, compliment the cute top. The distance of the Saturday run depends on marathon training plans. We could do the 12-mile flat Swamp Loop (yes, please!) or the punishing hills of the 15-mile Jacob's Ladder (groan). One of us will drop Gatorade and water the night before. Negotiations typically begin Friday night, via text message: "How far are we going tomorrow? What route should we run? What time can you start?"

We talk and talk and talk, about everything and nothing. It's amazing we don't run out of things to talk about.

With me hardly even noticing, she—and her family—gradually wove a tight web of support around my daughter and me that went way beyond running. She sent her husband over when the roof leaked, and when the pipes burst, and when the pull-out pantry cabinet fell off its track. They invited us over for afternoon BBQs and to her father-in-law's lake house in the summer. Her teenage kids gamely absorbed my younger-than-them daughter into their fold. My daughter and I were discussing our relationship with them one day, and she said they weren't exactly friends, they were more than that. "They're *framily*."

"Hi, friend." She was as welcoming at mile 23 of Boston as she'd been on every run during the past three years.

This was our third marathon together, which fortuitously landed during spring break, so our families came along. We did every long run together in preparation—through a record-setting cold, snowy winter—but we also readily agreed we'd each run our own race, as we had the previous two. "We each just run what's best and appropriate for each of us to get the most out of ourselves," Shalane had told me about her and Kara's race-day strategies. "I will train with you, and give you a hug and wish you well on the starting line, and mean it genuinely," said Kara. "But when the gun goes off, I'm not your friend. If I can stick it to you, I'm going to." Kara laughed, but also added: "I'll be your friend again at the finish." Fast Teacher Friend and I agreed with their philosophy—except the part where they run at a 5:30-per-mile pace.

We boarded a rickety and overheated school bus at the Boston Common to take us to the start in Hopkinton a good three hours before our race start, but the time passed quickly. We sipped water and nibbled on bagels and animal crackers and chatted nervously. We'd just enough time in the Athlete's Village to wait in porta-potty lines, shed our unnecessary layers of throw-away clothes, and walk together to our start corrals: hers ahead of mine because of her faster qualifying time. "Good-bye! Good luck! See you at the finish!" And she gave me, of course, a big, teacher-style hug.

The race was huge for a marathon—thirty-six thousand people—and also too warm. The temperature was a bright sixty-seven, but hot in the piercing spring sun—and given our 11 a.m. start, we'd be running through the heat of the day. I kept my eye on my watch, trying not to get carried away on the early downhill miles, and stuck to my plan of sipping Gatorade every 2 miles. Along the way, a running-club acquaintance fell in step with me for a few miles, but I wasn't in the mood to chat about my recent history. Indeed, I was annoyed—a sign, in retrospect, I was already getting dehydrated and cranky. Which is one of the reasons when I saw Fast Teacher Friend on the other side of the course around the halfway mark, I didn't make the effort to cross over and reach her.

So I passed Fast Teacher Friend, but I was running scared as the sun beamed down through leafless spring trees. How long could I hold her off? In the first marathon we'd run together, she'd started and stayed ahead of me the whole time, as expected. The second one was hot and humid, and she suffered more than me, so I passed her around mile 18, and finished slightly ahead; both of our times were slower than hoped. In Boston, it was brash (and foolish) of me to pass so early, and I ran knowing I should rein in my pace but also worrying the day was only growing warmer.

At mile 22 on the sidelines, I saw my daughter and Fast Teacher Friend's husband and kids. *Hello! Hello! Hello!* In their photos of me, which I'd see later, I look happy, if a little fried. But I could feel my pace falling off precipitously. I would also learn later that when she passed by our crew a few paces behind me, her husband had said, "Tish is just in front of you. GO GET HER!"

Hi, friend! We ran about half of a mile together to the next aid station, where we grabbed Gatorade to sip and water to pour on our heads. "How are you doing?" I asked. "Good!" she said, a little too enthusiastically. If her pace was falling off, it was not precipitously. I thought, *Wouldn't it be nice if I could keep up with her and finish the last 3 miles of the Boston Marathon together?*

I had nothing left, which is why my heart sank. She did and pulled away to finish 3 minutes ahead of me. In 3 miles. You don't have to be a teacher to do that math. Ouch.

After crossing the finish line, we wound our separate ways through Back Bay to our prear-ranged meeting spot in a hotel lobby to join our families, change clothes (no shower!), and make our way back to her car for the five-hour drive home. We both had to go to work the next day. We stopped for sandwiches along the way and bored our families with our mile-by-mile race recap. We were gritty, sticky, exhilarated. We'd done it—together!—the Boston Marathon.

What comes next for me? I'm still not sure. When you spend more than twenty years with one person, it takes a while to figure out. But one thing I am quite sure of: As I keep moving forward, I am grateful for every shared mile—with the fifty-stater, the ultrarunner, the triathlete, the social worker, the reluctant partner. And even if Fast Teacher Friend sprints—or shuffles—by me in the last miles of the next marathon, knowing she'll be there at the finish with a sweaty hug is comfort enough for now.

TAKE IT *From* A MOTHER
DOES YOUR FAMILY "GET" YOUR RUNNING?

*"My family knows running makes me happy and therefore
it benefits our family, but it is just my thing."*

—ALICIA (Her truth: "No matter how shitty the rest of my day—or life—feels, no one can take those 5 early morning miles away from me. And if I can run on a dark track at 6 a.m., there's nothing I can't do—or handle.")

"Not really. There is tolerance, but no real interest."

—SHARA (Adds: "Well, the kids are mildly curious.")

*"My immediate family gets it. My husband has started doing some running, and
my son joined the middle school cross-country team. My parents, however, don't
get it. They think running is bad for me and that I'm wasting my time, which gets
me down sometimes. I gave my mom a framed finisher photo from my first half-
marathon as a Christmas gift and she wouldn't even display it—yet she had holiday
cards from a politician and many photos of mysterious distant cousins' babies on
the fridge. I'm not sure why I crave their acceptance at age forty-two, but I do."*

—LISA (Sets annual running goals at her running group's December holiday party.)

*"My husband thinks running is crazy, but he is really awesome about
supporting me. He had a homemade breakfast waiting for me every
Saturday last summer when I got home from my long runs."*

—WENDY (Loves to do planks, hates to do squats.)

*"I feel very supported by my family and love, love, love when my
boys ask me, 'Did you run this morning, Mommy?' When they ask, it
sounds like, 'Did you save the world this morning, Mommy?'"*

—COLLEEN (Advice for beginners: "Nobody is watching or judging you. And if they are watching, they're thinking, 'Damn. That's what I should be doing.'")

"Overall, my family is good about it—my kids have done short races, and we travel to my races together. I have a stay-at-home husband, so I try not to be gone at work and also be gone for running. Sometimes my husband will mention running is selfish, but I tell him to feel free to get up at 5 a.m. for his 'me' time as well. That usually shuts him up."

—MELANIE (Secret weapon: Run no matter what. "So I'm tired. It's raining. I'm in a bad mood. Don't think about it; go run.")

"The kids get it, but my husband does not. Makes me feel lonely when no adult cares about my accomplishments. Then I guess that's what Facebook is for."

—LISA (Races every month. When a race was canceled because of a pending storm, she did 13.1 miles solo the day before.)

"Yes, hallelujah! My husband is just as addicted as I am. My parents are/were both successful runners. Same for my brother and sister. My kids think all mommies and daddies do it."

—MARTHA (Favorite workout? "Anything that's hard and with friends. Either a tempo run or track work.")

"My husband is a distance swimmer, so he gets it. He recently successfully swam the English Channel. I seem sane in comparison."

—JUDY (Came close to being hit by a car while running in Ireland. "He didn't use a turn signal, and I wasn't expecting him to be on that side of the road.")

"Yes, they totally get it because they have experienced my transformation, and they know what an important part running plays in my day-to-day life."

—MICHELLE (Lost 135 pounds with regular running and healthy eating.)

"They get that I like medals."

—LAURA (Perfect running weather + outfit: seventies, tank, shorts. "SoCal girl born and raised.")

TAKING THE LONG WAY HOME
by Heather Johnson Durocher

He handed the jewelry case to me unceremoniously—not cracked open, and certainly not as he knelt on one knee. We were standing in the infield of the high school track, surrounded by hundreds of shrieking, elementary school girls. Our two boys, ages eight and four, stood next to my husband, scanning the crowd for their older sister, one of the frenzied fourth-grade girls ready to run the Girls on the Run 5K, a race they'd been training for with my help for the past eight weeks.

I held the unopened box in my hand, knowing what was inside. I worked with a jeweler on the redesign of my wedding band and knew Joe, my husband of ten years, planned to pick it up earlier that day. I hadn't expected to receive it, though, just minutes before I'd be running 3.1 miles with more than eight-hundred elementary school girls. But I quickly pushed aside the *why now?* in favor of seeing the finished piece.

In hindsight, I would've preferred a less chaotic time—perhaps a quiet evening somewhere—for such a moment. Truthfully, though, Joe is a no-frills kind of guy, never one to make big romantic plans, especially when our marriage was pretty tender. Buying me a new ring was, on its own, a rather significant gesture for him. Our eyes met for a quick moment, before I glanced back at the box and opened it.

I've never been a woman who covets expensive jewelry, but I really had wanted this ring that was, as it happened, on the pricier side. It was more than simply a replacement for the original that had lost its one-carat center stone on a cold and snowy day months prior. The ring contained most everything its original did—six tiny diamonds, plus the center stone that had eventually been discovered stuck beneath a dirty floor mat in our Jeep—but also something more: renewed meaning to our then-fragile partnership. It was a chance to mend something broken, nearly lost.

Bling or no bling, it was a treat to have something so custom, something so *me*. As I turned the ring over in my hands, it felt both foreign and comfortable. It felt like hope.

Of course jewelry doesn't solve marital problems any more than popping an ibuprofen before a race cures a nagging injury. A decade into our marriage, I was smart enough to realize this when I slid the band on my ring finger that balmy May evening. But somehow a refurbished ring seemed appropriate to mark a fresh start after the ugliest years of our marriage.

The cloud appeared when Joe lost his job in late 2006, which led to weeks of wondering how we'd make ends meet, particularly given that we'd bought a new, larger house after the birth of

Alex, our third child, just one year earlier. Though many others would eventually lose their jobs in America's worst recession since the Great Depression, Joe's position was among the first wave of casualties. We felt alone among our friends.

Our marriage faltered as Joe, who had built successful businesses and had a tough time sitting still, grew depressed and angry. Admittedly, I didn't help matters. The circle of "friends" we had at the time weren't our people, though I pretended they were. Joe never fully took to their boating-and-golfing-and-cocktailing lifestyle but went along with it to appease me. I'd grown up middle-class like Joe but justified our involvement with these decidedly white-collar friends with the fact I'd connected with several of these women through exercise and our kids.

While I couldn't relate to taking off on frequent girls' trips, like long shopping weekends in Chicago, followed by couples-only spring breaks on exotic islands, these women encouraged me to sign up for my first race, a 25K, and five of us ran it together. I also spent many a summer afternoon with them, taking our kids to the beach, picking blueberries at a local farm, and just hanging out at one another's homes, talking books and cool new recipes to try as our kids played nearby. It was the first time I had connected with a group of women not only because our kids got along, but because we had things in common in addition to motherhood. I yearned for Joe to connect with their husbands, to join them mountain biking (he tried: the group was too competitive for him), or go on a golf outing (not a chance: no interest in making small talk with people with whom he had very little in common). I failed to see just how unhappy Joe was with these friends—and just how miserable he was with our life.

In fall 2007, I took an office job in public relations, after seven years of being a freelance writer. I exchanged a flexible schedule doing something I loved—writing for magazines, newspapers, and websites (and spending time with my three young children)—for a great salary and an office overlooking Lake Michigan. The job lasted only a year, but it was a complete disaster. Not only was the work mind-numbingly boring and required travel, it also led to something I never pictured happening: losing sight of myself and giving away my heart to another man. For months I had an affair with a guy who lived across the country—we'd met during a business trip—and as Joe and I floundered, I thought I'd found a safe place to sort everything out. *What was I doing working this job? What kind of mother was I now that I was no longer spending so much time with my kids? Could Joe and I even find our way back to each other if individually we were so frustrated and confused with where we had each ended up?*

I knew the affair was wrong. I could hardly stand the person I'd become when I allowed myself to really think about it, but I clung to this other person because he reminded me I was more than my circumstances. I could be more, be *better*. At the time, though, I had no idea what being better actually looked like.

That Joe and I were still together in May 2010 was nothing short of a miracle. We still didn't quite understand it ourselves sometimes, though we both shared with each other over and over that we didn't want to *not* be together. I often thought about something I read long ago, about long-term marriage: A man was asked how he and his wife managed to stay together for more than thirty years. His response: "We never wanted a divorce at the same time." As Joe and I reconciled, turning our focus back toward each other in a tentative, hopeful way—much like the way I return to running following an injury—I understood firsthand that wise perspective. At that point in our marriage, we'd ridden out the lowest lows of our union, and we'd definitely turned a very large corner. Still, we weren't sure about the road ahead.

I looked down at that ring multiple times that night of the Girls on the Run 5K, rubbing its smooth, squared side with my left thumb as I ran alongside my exuberant and tired team of young girls. The next morning, I found myself unconsciously toying with the ring, as I pushed myself hard in my city's annual Memorial Day weekend half-marathon to finish in 1:47:47, a new PR.

I'd been running for a few years at that point, and I'd experienced tangible, positive changes as a result—most notably a leaner and stronger body—but something intangible, something revelatory and significant was stirring within me. Each mile I logged, every race I completed, brought me closer to the realization I had gotten very good at self-sabotage and self-destruction. I was a champion at surrounding myself with the wrong people, at seeking validation outside of my marriage and family, at numbing myself with alcohol and cigarettes, to name a few. I didn't want to do any of that anymore.

That spring, when I got the new ring, life began to feel less hazy and complicated and more promising. I felt myself emerging from a fog that even a long run had a difficult time penetrating. Attempting a run hungover isn't ideal, I had learned, both physically and emotionally. My legs and lungs weren't up for the slog, but even more excruciating were the inner demons that came out in force when I headed out for these morning-after runs. As my feet pounded the ground, voices shouted, *Who do you think you are, trying to better yourself while still so clearly a hot mess? You're never going to get your act together, Heather!* Ultimately, I couldn't reconcile running toward a healthier life with staying up late to polish off "just one more" glass of wine. Eventually, finally, I stopped repeating the same mistake.

Joe and I spent more time together, quality time: We really listened to each other as we opened up and ignored what we began calling outside noise that most often came in the form of other people's thoughts about our life. We brought it all back to us, to our family of five, the most important thing to both of us. Instead of withdrawing (my natural inclination during conflict) or growing angry (Joe's first response), we decided the only way to make it through and to come out stronger together was to be real and honest. "I'm being vulnerable right now" was our new code phrase when one of us wanted to share something without fear of judgment. Perhaps for the first time in our marriage, we fully accepted each other and weren't taking the other for granted.

At the same time, I knew this mending of my marriage depended on tending to myself. The more honest I was with myself about how I'd hurt myself and my family with the choices I'd made, the stronger partner I became to Joe. I couldn't change Joe—that he had to do on his own—but I could alter my ways. Running propelled me in this direction.

The new ring was gorgeous, but it wasn't the greatest gift my husband gave me. Instead, as we forged a path of forgiveness and healing, the most important, bittersweet present Joe gave me was time to run and space to run far away from him. I was like a wound; I needed fresh air and time to heal, to find myself again.

In the months following that weekend of racing while wearing my new wedding ring, I was recommitted to my marriage, but I also had big plans. Plans that didn't involve Joe, or even the kids. My best running friend and I signed up to run a half-marathon thousands of miles away, in Eugene, Oregon, my first out-of-state race and the farthest I'd gone away from my family. It took place over Labor Day weekend, just a couple of days before school started. It was strange to leave my family behind, but it was mostly exhilarating. Reminding myself that running was making me a better person eased my mom guilt, especially as I stuffed my Brooks shoes into my carry-on bag and left for the airport to catch my flight to Oregon.

That November, there was the Hot Chocolate 15K in Chicago with another running friend, and not even a year later, a girls' weekend in San Francisco to run the Nike Women's Marathon. Somehow I squeezed in a trip to Boulder earlier that summer, too, where I attended a fitness bloggers' conference and ran for the first time at altitude, up into the Flatirons and through breathtaking canyons.

During this time Joe found work, sometimes a few different jobs cobbled together to make ends meet. I never doubted his work ethic, but I was floored by just how much he wanted to do right by our kids and by me. He tackled physically demanding jobs, like a short-term, on-call gig working for a funeral home that required frequent middle-of-the-night pickups from nursing homes and the hospital.

Sandwiched in between these work changes for Joe and all of my far-flung trips were hours-long trail runs for me near our home. I was also writing more about running, and meeting like-minded runners who inspired me to keep exploring this endurance lifestyle I'd clung to like a life preserver after falling overboard. Through it all, Joe surprised me with his acceptance of this new passion of mine. We missed each other—we'd talk and text frequently when I was away—but I also sensed he was discovering his own place within our newly defined marriage and family life. My traveling allowed him to connect with Emma, Andrew, and Alex in different ways. He was making meals and shuttling them to various activities, giving him lots of time to simply be with them.

There were tense moments for sure, when it all got to be too much and we'd fight about a place I wanted to go and how much it would cost. "But I'm doing something healthy, for me and for us," I'd say to him, urgently. "I'm a happier person when I run. I'm a better person for you, for our kids." He couldn't argue this point, and he couldn't even say I didn't sometimes invite him to come along with me. I wanted him to join me on the trip to Colorado, which would've been good for us: a short mountain getaway without kids. But he was still working things out for himself and was focused on keeping things humming for us financially. Most importantly, he was in the midst of starting a new business, one that made him happier than I'd seen him in a long time.

I also think he just wasn't there yet, wasn't ready to enter my new world. I know it was hard for him to watch me change and grow, even if it meant I was a better Heather, because he had to let the old Heather go a little for it to happen.

It all was so thrilling and healing, this newfound passion for health I'd unearthed. Yet I look back now and I am humbled, and maybe even a little embarrassed, at how entrenched I became in *me*, in getting over the person I no longer wanted to be, the woman who had caused so much heartache and nearly got divorced. I was unselfish, but also kind of selfish. Balancing the need to be good to yourself with the responsibilities of doing the right things is a more complicated act than I expected.

As I trained for my first marathon in the winter of 2010–11, my running coach and friend, Lisa, told me the late Dr. George Sheehan used to say we're all "an experiment of one." You can follow a training plan and take great advice, she told me, but you also need to be aware of how your own body responds, then adjust accordingly. Once you really start looking at these things on an individual basis, it's remarkable how in tune you can get with yourself. You find out chocolate gel agrees best with your stomach. You learn two marathons in one year are just too much, leaving you prone to injuries. That eating oatmeal and sipping just a tiny bit of coffee before a race revs you up in all the right ways.

As the weeks of aiming for 26.2 miles unfolded and I pushed through training days on cold, snowy mornings, I realized this thinking could be applied to my marriage as well, and to all aspects of my life, actually. I might think a friend's marriage or family or job is pretty special, but I no longer look to it as the example to which I should model my own life. I realized I don't know anyone else's intimate life any better than they know mine. Instead I need to focus on me, and on what works for my marriage, my important relationships, and the life I've built. A long-distance affair doesn't make anything better, and neither does denying my marriage needs help.

These days, I'm proud of just how far I've come—and how far Joe and I have progressed together. We have stumbled and fallen and gotten back up . . . and fallen again before righting it yet one more time. I embrace my imperfect life, in no small part because of my discovery of running and all it has brought into my life. Nearly everything I know about myself—the person I am today at forty—I've discovered through running.

Through miles and miles, I've processed and reflected and thought and dreamed in entirely eye-opening and (sweat-drenched) cleansing ways. I ran and raced and stood in awe of my leaner, stronger legs and of my cleared, focused mind. I brought this all back to my marriage. I realized I could run hard and I could love hard. I could stick with a training plan and reach a race goal, and I could hope for a better marriage and do the work of strengthening our relationship. I could be kinder to myself, and we could become better partners to each other.

And something interesting happened along the way: Joe entered my world, as have our kids. Even though they were always active themselves, my family suddenly was just *there*. Cheering me on at mile 21 of my first marathon, navigating Boston's public transit (and ridiculous, record-breaking heat) to find a spot at mile 24 of my toughest and most memorable 26.2, and going along with my camping-at-state-parks-so-I-can-run-them-and-blog-about-it plan I hatched one summer. Our family of five has run numerous 5Ks, most memorably a humid July race in our hometown that marked Alex's first race at age seven. ("I can just throw it down on the ground?" he asked incredulously after stopping at an aid station and watching runners ditch their water cups.) Joe, who ran his first half-marathon in 2013, trained with our twelve-year-old Andrew for a 10K together.

If running and training and racing have taught me nothing else, it is time and hard work and patience—sometimes excruciating patience—yield satisfying and sweet returns, both in life and running.

Despite being four years old, my reworked wedding ring still feels new. It's my daily reminder of what I came so close to losing, yet was somehow able to keep. I can still hear Andrew's breathless words from the back seat of the Jeep many moons ago: *"Mom, I think I just found the diamond that fell out of your ring!"*

I'd lost the diamond from my original wedding ring a week earlier, rushing home after a harried day. Once I realized it was probably gone forever, I substituted my grandmother's amethyst ring as my wedding band. That purple-stoned ring was pretty, but I'd wondered if Joe and I, muddling through those dark days of our marriage, would ever do something about a new wedding band.

Seeing that diamond, that precious stone given by a handsome guy to a young woman a lifetime ago, brought tears to my eyes. It could have fallen out anywhere, been swept away in myriad directions. And yet it had been there all along. It only needed to be found.

TAKE IT *From* A MOTHER
IS BALANCE ACHIEVABLE IN LIFE AS A MOTHER RUNNER?

"Yes, if you know you can't have it all at once. I think life comes in stages, and you can have everything you want . . . just not all at the same time."

—ANDREA (Toenails on her second toes are always black.)

"A work mentor pointed out that just because something is balanced doesn't mean the scales are even. Sometimes, one scale has more weight— and needs more attention—than the others. I try to keep that in mind. Sometimes it's work; sometimes it's my son; sometimes it's my marriage; sometimes it's my training. Doesn't mean I am out of balance."

—ANDREA (Runs with her big German shepherd. "People cross the street to avoid us.")

"I don't think balance exists. I think life is a constant state of overbalancing in whatever direction is most important and most necessary in that moment, then readjusting in the other directions as necessary. Running has taught me you can have a constant theme, though, and return to it as a way to ground yourself, even if you can't do all things all the time."

—ALISON (A picture of her daughter wearing her running shoes was her phone's wallpaper during the NYC Marathon. "Every time I needed a little boost, I'd look at it.")

"Only if you have a partner who is supportive and gives you the time it takes to train and go to races."

—MARJORIE (Her running is "steady, therapeutic, and joyful.")

"Total balance? No. But I don't know if there's ever total balance in the life of a mother, runner or not."

—AMY (Running brought her "out of my shell, which I've lived in for so long. I feel like I have a community to which I belong for the first time ever.")

"Really tough one! I'm finding that, as women, it's really difficult to have it all. We come to a crossroads in life where we decide whether to pursue a more successful career or start a family. It's hard to give 100 percent to both, so you always end up sacrificing—even if it's just a little bit—on one of them. It's similar with running. You have to give something up to make the time to run, maybe an extra hour of sleep or watching a movie with your kids."

—ERIN (Only runs on a treadmill if she's staying in a hotel.)

"Yes. It's hard and takes a lot of patience and planning, but it's possible. Also, we need to be flexible and forgiving. I tell myself, even if I only got 5 miles in for a week, it's still 5 miles. Next week will be better."

—KATE (Ran her first 50K in March. "I trained for it outside through a tough Iowa winter. I'll never do that again.")

"Balance could be achievable for some, but I think as women we all put way too much pressure on ourselves to perform at the highest level for everything we do. I really want to eliminate the word 'just' from my vocabulary so I can stop saying I 'just' ran the half-marathon, not the full marathon."

—DONNA (Had a deer run into her once. "It was very creepy; I can still remember the feel of the deer's short hair and strong body.")

"Yes. I have two boys, ages two and five. I work full time. I run. Everyone gets the same amount of time; you choose how to spend it."

—KATIE (Strategy for stinky running clothes: "When it doubt, throw it out.")

"Yes. The bottom line for me is knowing when to say no."

—MARY (Started running at age forty "to see if I could.")

"If balance is achievable as a mother, I missed the memo."

—LAVON (Made her own version of a marathon-pace bracelet; instead of mile splits, she had a name of somebody special in her life and dedicated the mile to them.)

RUNNING APART
by Jennifer Graham

My husband didn't run when we were married, and far as I know, he doesn't run now that we're divorced.

This isn't *why* we're divorced, mind you. The separation agreement says nothing about running—or the lack thereof. When we stood before the judge, and muttered consent that we were "irreparably broken" despite eighteen years and four kids, we were talking about the marriage, not my heart-rate monitor.

In fact, we never talked about my heart-rate monitor at all.

So when you survey the carcass of my marriage, which strode boldly for fifteen years before developing a debilitating and ultimately fatal limp, you are entirely right to ask, *Well, wasn't that a problem?*

I know. I've asked that myself. *If a heart-rate monitor matters to one spouse, shouldn't it matter to both?* Can a marriage or partnership thrive and endure if one person runs, and the other one doesn't?

There are two schools of thinking. The first is the School of Opposites Attract, attended by those who believe Yin loves Yang precisely because Yang is so different from Yin. These relationships work, the thinking goes, because the lovers complement each other, adding richness and depth and variety to each other's lives. Also, bringing a fan club.

It's hard to be slavishly adoring of someone who does exactly the same things you do. If, for example, you have just returned from running 10 miles in a freakin' blizzard, you are much more likely to find someone waving palm branches and singing hosanna if he is a sedentary schlub who has to hoist himself off the couch to put on the parade. Also, somebody's got to watch the kids while you're at the Turkey Trot, and it's grievously hard to find a babysitter on Thanksgiving, particularly one who will make the gravy while he's watching the kids.

So, yes, there are benefits to being a runner in a relationship with a non-runner.

But there's another school, and it is the School of Like Attracts Like. Those who matriculate there understand the importance of tribe, the pleasures and comfort derived from nesting with someone who looks, thinks, and smells vaguely like you. And if he exercises like you, all the better, for he will know what questions to ask. My husband, the non-runner, didn't. To be fair, he tried; he really did. At least before the limp made us both stumble so often and so catastrophically.

I was a runner for three years already when we started dating, so he signed on to life with a runner—albeit a fat, slow one—and I think he really believed he was my number one fan.

When I returned from a run, he would always ask, in varying degrees of earnestness, "How was your run?" and I think he considered himself nurturing and caring. But because he didn't run and had no desire to, he didn't understand "How was your run?" wasn't enough. Not nearly.

Here is what I wanted him to ask, even when I didn't know it at the time: *How far did you run? How fast did you go? How was your breathing? Did your legs feel strong? Have you recovered yet from Sunday's long run? How is that little ache in your hamstring? What is your Powersong on your Nike Plus? Did you see any deer in the woods? Did you step over any snakes? Water, GU, or Gatorade? Did you run any negative splits?*

Okay, maybe we shouldn't have talked about negative splits.

But we should have talked about heart-rate monitors.

He should have known how important having one was to me.

Here's how I got mine.

One year, I started dropping hints in January about the Polar S410 I'd been eyeing.

Did I *need* a heart-rate monitor? Of course not. I am a recreational runner, badass only in my own mind. But I'd been running for nigh-on twenty years, and have the heart of a runner, if not the shape. Which is to say, I always want to be faster and fitter.

A heart-rate monitor, I thought, would help me.

So I dropped lots of hints, to which he seemed receptive, so much so that I even told my best friend I was getting a heart-rate monitor for Valentine's Day.

But then Valentine's Day came, and there were . . . flowers.

Roses, yes, and with chocolate and dinner and a Vermont Teddy Bear. It was all as expensive as a heart-rate monitor. It's not that he was cheap. But what my heart wanted, my heart didn't get. And so, the next month, I got a heart-rate monitor from someone else.

He was a guy I'd been dating, although I didn't know it at the time. Married people don't "date," at least not people other than their spouses. But they do "have lunch" and "exchange e-mails," and if they're not careful, even if they don't break any commandments, they can irreparably break each other's hearts and a marriage or two in the process.

So yeah—of course, you see this coming—this guy was a runner.

Not only did he run, but he was also a hardcore cyclist. He had once ridden his bike through three states, and he had biceps that could make a non-sedentary-type of girl like me all tingly.

The talented writer and runner Rachel Toor once penned an essay for *Running Times* magazine called "Speed Goggles: Why Fast Men Make the Heart Beat Quicker." It was about her search for a STYF man. STYF: smarter, taller, younger, and faster. "Speed goggles" was her riff on "beer goggles": the thing you don when you've had too much to drink and everything you view is distorted. "I know lots of great and handsome men who slog through marathons at a slow and steady pace," Toor wrote. "It's not that I wouldn't go out with them, but when I see the cadaverous guys striding out before the gun goes off, my heart begins to race."

I got that. I so got that.

I did not want a cadaverous guy—if I accidentally rolled over him during the night, I might kill him—but I understood Toor's longing for an athletic man who matched her ability, or at the very least, challenged her, and admired her stride.

And thought she needed a heart-rate monitor.

So, as you might imagine, all this—the marriage, my affair—ended badly. I do not ask for forgiveness, or even sympathetic clucking. Years have passed, and I have come to grips with being not a good example, but a horrible warning. My warning is this: Sometimes it doesn't matter if you run and your partner doesn't.

Sometimes it does.

You can't always figure this out until it's over, when you look back and see how you were running apart as fast as you could, confidently, blindly, stupidly, perhaps. And your heart-rate monitor—damn it, it's never worked quite right—did not beep shrilly to tell you this. Eventually, you come to, a zillion miles from home, and contemplate the loneliness of the long-distance mother, and decide that it is not good, and you want to go elsewhere, to enroll in another school.

Then, what you get is a negative split.

You will survive it, yes. You will survive it because you are a badass and you can run 10 miles (*10 miles!*) in a blizzard, and you do it, not for adulation, but because it's Who You Are. You will survive it because you are a runner, and while bells and whistles are nice, you do not *need* a heart-rate monitor or even someone to give you a heart-rate monitor. All you need is a path on which to run like Thoreau: confidently, in the direction of your dreams. (And it helps if your resting heart rate is in the low fifties.)

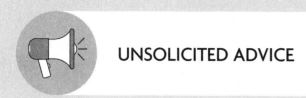

UNSOLICITED ADVICE

While pregnant women are the biggest—both in numbers and, ahem, size—receivers of unsolicited advice, mothers with young children are a close second.

"Should you have her here?" I, Dimity, remember an older lady asking me while I strolled a screaming Amelia, two weeks old, through the grocery store. I probably just nodded, but I really wanted to say: "This child is sucking the life out of me, I have one slimy cucumber in my produce drawer, my husband is back at work, my mom left yesterday so I cried for two hours, and my breakfast this morning was a stale chocolate chip cookie. So, yes, I should have her here."

Whoa. Didn't realize that encounter struck such a deep nerve.

Anyway, people naturally want to tell you what to do. Mother runners are no different, but the good news is the following advice, all in one-sentence, easy-to-retain bits, is actually truly helpful. (And if it's not, well, just smile politely and keep pushing your cart along.)

PERSPECTIVE

"No disclaimers allowed: You run; you are a runner."

—MARNI (Hasn't lost any weight since she started running. "But my masseuse told me I'm all muscle. That's got to count for something, right?")

"It will get easier, but it will never be easy."

—KATIE (PS "You will get faster, but never as fast as you would like to go.")

"How you want to feel is your choice."

—CYNDI (Feels so good after morning run in the summer, she wants to jump her husband. "Do endorphins really work like that?" *Blushing*.)

"Some days are going to suck."

—CHRISTINE (Her abs are six-pack, but she stores them in "a soft-sided cooler.")

"Don't make it so complicated or worrisome that running becomes just one more thing to drive you crazy."

—TINA (Loves running because "even though I'm not very fast, most of the time I feel like I'm flying.")

"A run might have been shorter or slower or felt harder than what you had planned, but it was better than no run at all."

—MEGAN (While training for longer races, wakes in the middle of the night thinking, *Oh, man, I have an eleven-miler in just three hours!* "Intimidates the crap out of me.")

"Pedicures never look sexy when you don't have all your toenails."

—KELLY (When injured, she "lifts heavy things and gets in cardio any way I can.")

"Running is much more fun when you have someone to chat with during the miles."

—ADRIENNE (Says her brain is the weakest part of her body. "I'm not sure I'll ever stop doubting my abilities, but I'll never give up trying.")

"Running is like saving money for retirement. You should invest regularly to get interest and benefits for life."

—CHRISTINE (She's a family doctor with an obstetrical practice, so she gets two sentences.)

"When you don't want to run, put on your gear, then go stand outside or on the treadmill and determine if you feel a spark; only after you do this are you excused from not running."

—KATHY (Got that advice when she had a hard time motivating *herself* after her mom died.)

"You only get one 'first' for all of your running milestones, so be proud of yourself."

—KAREN (Loves watching others reach their goals. "It's like after you become a parent, you realize Christmas is so much more fun when you give gifts to your kids instead of receiving them.")

"*Uno mas*: one more mile, one more run, one more (whatever) is possible."

—ERIKA (Gets in her runs at lunchtime. "I can get in 4 miles, change, and make it back to my desk in an hour. I might be sweaty and gross, but I feel great.")

"Don't let outdated beliefs about yourself keep you from moving beyond yourself."

— LINDSAY (Start a crockpot meal and throws a load of laundry into the washing machine before she heads out on a weekend long run to feel like she's helping around the house.)

"Breathe and believe."

—SARAH ("Two wagging tails" make her feel guilty when she's not up for a run.)

"*Kia kaha*."

—JILL (Translation: a Maori phrase for "stay strong.")

"If I can do it, you can do it."

—CHRISTINE (An ex-smoker who started running at age forty-four. Still, "I'd rather clean my house than go for a run.")

GEARING UP

"Get thee to a running-shoe store and get properly fit."

—JESSICA (Proudest running moments: when friends ask her for advice.)

"At least once a week, leave your watch at home, then run as far and as fast or as slow as you feel like going."

—COURTNEY (Seems to pick up race hitchhikers. "I am good at keeping a steady pace, and more races than not, somebody runs a few steps off my shoulder. Sometimes they ask if it's okay, and sometimes they're just like race stalkers.")

"Buy an awesome bra that costs three to four times what you think a bra should cost."

—JENNIFER (At the end of the run, when all she wants to do is quit, she tells herself to run to a tree. "Then I do it: not run *nearly* to the tree or *almost* to the tree. TO. THE. TREE.")

"Don't wear cotton underwear."

—CARLY (On a long run in the middle of nowhere, she pooped her capris. "My mom had to pick me up. I rode home sitting on a trash bag, then threw out the capris.")

TRAINING

"Figure out what parts of running—morning or night, solo or group, trail or road—work for you, then organize your training accordingly."

—KRISTIN (Describes her running as crucial "to me and those who live with me.")

"Don't miss more than two days of workouts in a row."

—LEANNE (Gauges her effort by the amount of urine leakage. "I've had three kids; if I'm leaking in a race, then I am running hard enough!")

"Commit to three days a week of running and stick with it."

—KELLY (Her eleven-year-old has come within 7 seconds of her 5K PR of 22:38.)

"Running six days a week will break you."

—MICHELLE (PS "I seem to be especially injury-prone if I run more than four days a week with any amount of speedwork in the mix.")

"Run for minutes, not speed or distance."

—MEGAN (After a sprained ankle and bloody knee, her husband suggested she get a human-sized hamster ball to run in. "Not helpful.")

"Heed the 10 percent rule: Don't increase your mileage by more than 10 percent from one week to the next."

—MICHELLE (Does two 4-mile stints on the treadmill—"love the child care at the gym"—and one outdoor run weekly.)

"Learn to breathe in through your nose and out through your mouth."

—NIKKI (Breath point number two: When you have a side stitch, focus on breathing out when landing on the opposite foot of the side stitch. "I swear, it works.")

"To improve, push just the tiniest bit past your limit."

—AMANDA (Because of tornado warnings, she was pulled from the course of the Nashville Marathon at mile 20. Eight days later, she traveled to the Jersey Shore to finish her 26.2. "I started crying even before I crossed the finish line.")

"Find a song with a beat you can run to easily, and hang out in that rhythm."

—SHAWNEE (When she started running, she went with her dog. "If I got tired, I could just pretend I was walking the dog.")

"If you want to run faster, you have to run faster."

—JENNY (Advice giver: best running friend's husband, whose cross-country team won a national championship.)

"Do tempo runs on the treadmill: Run hard or fall off!"

—CYNDIE (If I weren't a runner, I'd be . . . "There are too many words to use here, and none of them are positive.")

"Don't race your training runs."

—KAREN (Not a fan of inclement weather. "I hate cold, am a wind wimp, and while I love heat for everything else in life, I don't deal well with it as a runner.")

"You can't save the effort you've put in and return a month—or weeks—later and be at the same place."

—ROBIN (Even though she thinks they're "disgusting," she eats a protein bar after long runs.)

"Your body is willing to go longer and farther than your head is."

—DEBRA (Not unrelated, her running motto is from Hebrews 12:1: "Let us run with perseverance the race that is set before us.")

"Just because something works for someone else, doesn't mean it's right for you."

—SYBIL (Hates lunges. "I am very tall and tippy and extremely inflexible.")

"It's okay to walk."

—JULIE (Reminds herself nobody—that she knows of anyway—has fallen asleep during a run. "So no matter how tired I feel, I can still get out there.")

"Elbows back and shoulders down."

—ANGELA (An important milestone in her running life: hiring a babysitter to come at 7 a.m. so she could run 8 miles in eight-degree weather.)

"Strength train, strength train, strength train."

> —TINA (During her first half-marathon, told herself to "GO!" at mile 12. "I ran my fastest mile and even got another woman to sprint with me! I yelled at her like a drill sergeant.")

"Walk backwards for one-hundred meters or so after a run to prevent shin splints."

> —CHRISTY (Got this advice in high school, and does it to this day, "even though I get weird looks when around other people.")

"Your knee problems probably aren't even in your knees and can usually be fixed with a foam roller."

> —CHLOE (She and her husband finished the *Runner's World* Holiday Run Streak. "It was hard and mostly annoying, but we are proud.")

"Rest and recovery are as important to a training plan as any individual run is."

> —AMY (Plays "Mama Said Knock You Out" by LL Cool J before every race.)

"The training is the work; the race is the party."

> —EMILY (Main goal: not walking during runs because, "I'm a masochist, solidly midwestern, and deeply fear being lazy.")

ON THE STARTING—AND FINISH—LINE

"Only race against yourself."

> —AUTUMN (Proudest running moment: breaking 30 minutes in a 5K. "I really trained, and it worked!")

"Don't minimize your victories."

> —MARY (Cross-trains by taking kettlebell class, playing soccer, and strength training.)

"If the body's healthy and well trained, and the heart is willing, the mind is the only thing standing in the way of a successful race."

> —LIA (Uses a rolling pin as her foam roller.)

"Work hard at the end of a race, not at the starting line."

—ABBI (Her husband's ex-wife complimented her strong legs. "Yeah . . . that was a good day.")

"If you are relaxed, happy, and focused, the PR will come."

—CAROLINE (Split her favorite capris during a Tough Mudder race—and shed tears. "Not because my arse was hanging out, but because I wrecked my favorite pants.")

"Everybody in fourth place and below gets the same medals."

—BECCA (Her sweaty, out-of-breath, victorious feelings after a morning run "set the tone for the whole day.")

"It helps to smile. (Really!)"

—PAULA (In her 5K PR, she pushed so hard she threw up in her mouth a few times—presumably when she wasn't smiling.)

"Focus on how you feel, not how you—or others—look."

—NORAH (Started running at age thirteen. "My parents said 'pick a sport,' and my mom said I could quit if I didn't like it. She lied.")

"Get enough sodium during long races."

—LAURA (While at the podiatrist for plantar fasciitis, "he took one look at the Old Navy flip-flops I was wearing and said he knew what the problem was.")

"Use your arms."

—HEATHER (Signed up for the Big Sur Marathon, knowing the cut-off for this [much tougher] course was 3 minutes faster than her time at the San Diego Rock 'n' Roll Marathon. She trained hard for six months, and beat the cutoff by 39 minutes.)

"Run the first half with your head, the third fourth with your legs, and the final fourth with your heart."

— KAT (At age twelve, started running from "the chaos at home and my nerdy seventh-grade haircut that marked me as an outcast.")

"Listen to your body during training; ignore it during a race."

> — KELLI (Makes her running mixes with her eleven-year-old son, then picks up the pace when one of his crazy rap/pop songs comes on.)

"When you're going for a PR, accept it's going to hurt and focus on a strategy to deal with—not fight—the pain."

> —MICHELLE (Has lowered her half-marathon PR from 2:14 to 1:37.)

"Your own race at your own pace."

> —JACKY (Her goal paces: 10K in less than an hour; half in 2:15; full in less than five hours.)

"Nobody but you cares about your race times."

> —JANA (Likes running along the river and filling out spreadsheets with her workouts.)

"Rest one day per mile after a hard race."

> —LAURA (Tries not to discuss PRs with her younger, *faster* sister.)

"Be proud of any finish: You're always faster than the people watching."

> —DENISE (Started running "to see what all the fuss was about.")

04

JOY:
Open Heart and Light Legs

"I love the quiet mornings in the subdivision. I live in Los Angeles, and weekend mornings are the best. The sun is starting to peek out, the birds are singing. The world is peaceful, if just for a moment.

—MARCI

RUNNING WITH *JO-EEY*

by Kristin Armstrong

"I'll be happy when . . ."

That sentiment worms into our society—and our heads—like an '80s song.

I'll be happy when I . . . graduate, find a job, have a boyfriend, buy a house, get a new car, get engaged, lose ten pounds, get married, get pregnant, have a baby, sleep through the night, go on vacation, lose ten pounds again, get a better job, send the kids to college, get an even better job, retire.

You know the drill, because it has been drilled into you.

Fleeting and unreliable, happy is such a fickle little bitch. Not unlike the "friend" you had in high school who would always ditch you if she got a date or an offer to do something more fun than watch movies and order pizza at your house. Happiness is based on circumstances and moods, timing and luck; as such, you have very little control over when that "friend" shows up, or how long she stays.

Even though I rationally know how elusive happiness is, I, like many people, was consumed with chasing it, like a boy on a playground. Happiness was the slippery measure of my success.

Like any addiction, unhealthy reliance on happiness causes too-crazy highs and too-blue lows. I became obsessed with getting the *I'll-be-happy* thing, eventually captured it, realized it didn't make me happy, sped by it and focused on the next thing I thought I needed to feel happy. It's the treadmill workout that is never complete, an endless repetitive effort that doesn't actually go anywhere.

I have a running coach named Gilbert Tuhabonye, who is a survivor of genocide in Burundi, Africa. His skin is covered in burn marks and machete scars, and he has the biggest, whitest smile: a shining beacon in his beautiful darkness. Running with Gilbert was the thing that finally kicked my happiness addiction. It was the result of many miles under the wisdom of his wings, but one incident stands out clearly in my memory.

One morning out on the Austin High School track, I am doing drills with my training group. I joke about being the caboose of the group, but I really don't mind it. Regardless of the arena, I prefer to surround myself with people more skilled than myself. But it can also be disheartening at times, watching these lean, leggy, more experienced people do something so well, so fast, so seemingly effortlessly while I huff and puff and work my ass off for such mediocre times, comparatively speaking.

Spring has sprung in Austin. The humidity causes sweaty, wayward layers to frizz out of my tangled ponytail and stick to the sides of my face. I gear up to do a series of 400s. I'm not really in the mood, but I'm trying to will myself, as if on a blind date: *Maybe this one will be the one?*

As usual, I am obsessing over my watch. *I'll be happy when . . .* I have a certain time in mind for my 400-meter intervals. Gilbert must read something in my face. "Kiki, forget the watch," he says in his Burundi accent. (I wish I could do it for you.) "Take it off. Today I want you to run with joy." He says "joy" lyrically, with two syllables: *jo-eey.*

I reluctantly undo the plastic strap on my Garmin and set it down on the bench next to the water jug and cone-shaped paper cups. I feel a bit awkward, almost naked. I am so accustomed to looking at the other runners, then looking down at my watch, measuring, rating, and berating myself. Now I just have an empty wrist. I line up behind the thoroughbreds, giving them their space. My first lap is self-conscious. I try too hard at the beginning and can't hold my pace around the final curve. The Thoroughbreds were already starting to go again as I sputter in.

"Bettah," Gilbert says, "Don't worry about everyone else. Run your own lap. Like you are alone on a beautiful morning. Find joy, like a child. Forget everything else."

I decide not to tell him that as a child in the morning, I would have more likely had my butt planted in front of the television, watching cartoons and eating handfuls of Froot Loops directly out of the box. I tuck my wet layers behind my ears. I notice everything: the pack ahead of me on the other side of the track; the scoreboard, with white letters across the top: NO EXCUSES: DO THE WORK; the unmotivated teenage P.E. class doing halfhearted calisthenics near the gym. I look down at my shoes, dirty from a recent rain.

And then I look straight ahead, take a deep breath, and stop noticing everything else. A pleasant calm comes over me. The Froot Loop kid is simply going for a spin. No big deal. I start out like Baby Bear's porridge: not too hot, not too cold. Juuuuust right. I don't look at my wrist, not once. I just run. I feel myself smiling, picking up speed instead of wearing out. I picture myself like Forrest Gump as a boy, running down the long driveway, his wooden braces breaking apart and flying off as he ran.

By the time I notice anything else again, I am crossing the line and Gilbert is screaming for me, jumping and flailing his arms as I finish. "You ran fasta' than ever befo'! You found jo-ey!" He hugged me.

I want to cry, doubled over, panting, about to barf. The race horses pat my sweaty back and murmur nice things into the humid air around me. It doesn't matter at all I didn't measure up to their best, because at last I am embracing my own.

I finally got the difference between happiness and joy; I felt it from the inside, springing up and bubbling from my own source. I had to stop looking out and start looking in. It isn't the discovery that running a 400 at a certain pace yields joy; it's the realization that joy can yield a different pace. It's less like trying harder and more like doing the work and then, at some point, simultaneously going for it and letting go. I had to shake off my measurements, my inner critic, my comparisons, and my relentless, fruitless perfectionism. In other words, I had to outrun my *happy-when* mentality in order to embrace my joy.

It took an African man, burned, scarred, forgiving, and free, to teach this whiny white girl a thing or two about joy. "Run with Joy" is Gilbert's mantra, motto, and motivation. Joy permeates every single thing he does, and emanates from every pore of who he is. Perhaps, when we are open and susceptible, joy is contagious. I definitely caught it that Tuesday morning.

I cool down on the grass on the perimeter of the track, blades of just-mowed green grass sticking to my shoes and calves. I think about how removing my watch is a metaphor for setting myself free, unhinging myself from outcomes, people and things I couldn't control, and rooting myself—and rooting for myself—in the present moment. The experience had way bigger implications for me than running a decent 400; it made sense in all areas of my life. Unnecessary striving and hyper-focus on outcomes is a killjoy.

More thoughts started collecting, the blessed clarity born of endorphins and the completion of effort. If happiness is external, joy is internal. If happiness is based on circumstance, joy is a baseline. If happiness is acquired, joy is bestowed. If happiness is a result of exertion, joy is a consequence of peace. If happiness is in what you do, joy is inherent in who you are. If happiness is an absence of pain or discomfort, joy is in its acceptance and integration. If happy *happens when*, joy exists in perpetuity behind the scenes.

Running was the catalyst for a distinction I desperately needed. Instead of aiming for happiness, I was now going to welcome joy into my life as often as possible. My Happy-When can turn into Joy-Now. Not complacent, but content. There is a difference.

When I look back, I realize running had been trying to teach me this for many years. A jiggly, leaky, excruciating postpartum run. A heaving, triple-jogger run to find some sanity. A who-the-hell-am-I-anymore-anyway, mother-of-toddlers run. An oh-shit-my-life-is-falling-apart run. A divorce recovery run: *If I can run x miles, I can do everything else ahead of me.* Marathon training runs that seemed to last all day. Ultramarathon training runs that seemed to last for days on end. My-teenage-kids-are-making-me-crazy reset runs. Runs jet-fueled by breakup misery. Solidarity runs beside a grieving friend. I was always running, but never running away; I was always running toward.

All of it, every single mile, was bringing me from there to here, teaching me joy, the best part, exists right here, right now. Even when running or marriage or motherhood—three things that can wear your ass out—seem unbearably hard, there is always a piece of joy to uncover. Right here. Right now.

TAKE IT *From* A MOTHER
IS THERE A SPIRITUAL SIDE TO YOUR RUNNING?

"During my first leg at Ragnar Northwest Passage, I ran down a mountain and passed a glistening lake. Never had I seen such beauty—until my third and final leg, a very difficult leg that had a significant climb through trees so tall I was beyond dwarfed. Their majesty and steadfastness through time struck a chord in me, and I realized how blessed I was to be able to run and have that experience. That run changed me forever. I now don't take any of my surroundings for granted. I offer up each run as a prayer of thanksgiving.

—DANIELLE (Has to match the colors of her socks, sports bra, headband, Nuun. "I have had terrible runs when I didn't care about what I wore.")

"I've found there is a very strong connection between being physically fit and spiritually fit. Not that all fit people are spiritual, and not that all spiritual people are fit. But I believe revelation for me and my family comes to me better when I am in better shape."

—GINA (Listens to gospel music on runs. "I love '80s music, but lyrics about sex and drugs while I'm running depress me.")

"There is a spiritual side to me, but I haven't run enough to claim there is—or isn't—a spiritual side to my running. I do run with gratitude."

—MARGIE (When she's "plodding along, or my joints ache from extra weight, I think of all I have to be grateful for, including the fact I haven't given up.")

"Oh, yes. I pray a lot when I run. It's time with me and God. Just us. How awesome!"

— MARY (Her husband often accuses her of running for an hour a day. "Oh, how I wish!")

"Running strengthens my soul as much as it strengthens my body."

—BRENDA (At a recent marathon, ran into her high school country-country teammate who she hadn't seen for twenty years. "I got to mile 25, and there was Jen, and I gave her a big hug. After the race, she said it was just what she needed at mile 25.")

"A lot of my running identity came about when I discovered my husband was experiencing an addiction, and the hurt and betrayal of the addiction was eating me alive. Running without music while training for a marathon saved me. The silence and stillness allowed me to really open up my heart in prayer. I was able to offer my tears and pain to the universe on those empty country roads, and I still feel a great deal of peace when I run in those places."

—KEIGHTY (Currently has three kids, a husband in school, and a full-time job. "I tell myself my running is perfect for where I am right now. I don't run to earn a cape.")

"No, but I always feel more in tune with myself, my body, and my mind after a run."

—JULIE (Has run the Bolder Boulder 10K eighteen times. In 1998, set PR of 49:50, and ran 50:10 in 2012. "I'm a smarter, more fit runner now.")

"My dad, a huge supporter of my running, died suddenly, and now I know he's with me every step of the way on my races and training runs. This year, Yom Kippur fell on a Saturday. I wrote to Another Mother Runner to get advice on how to deal with this. My dad was very traditional, and I know my dad would say (along with other mother runners), 'Get your a\$\$ to Temple.' I thought long and hard and decided this year my long run WAS my Temple. I chatted the entire time with my dad and felt an unbelievable sense of clarity."

—ILYCE (At mile 12 of that run, she found a magnet with the serenity prayer on it. "That was all I needed to know Dad was with me and I had made the right choice.")

"Definitely. When I started training, I'd start my run/walk with a prayer for friends, family, or people in need and think about them on my miles. I still do that. Selfishly, it motivates me. I stay committed to myself by honoring others."

—DENISE (Has a new definition for the iliotibial band acronym (ITB): "It's That Bad.")

"I run along Lake Michigan and get to witness that body of water through every season/storm/state of weather. It never ceases to be a spiritual experience for me to witness this Great Lake as I sweat it out. It often feels as though the sun, sky, water, and waves speak to me and encourage me along the way."

—CHRISTINE (Her first marathon was a trail marathon. "Not the best decision ever.")

RECIPE FOR DOUBLE DIGITS
by Adrienne Martini

Here is how you run 10 miles:

Wake up on the first day of spring, roll into your running gear, and wander downstairs for a snack before setting out.

Notice the outside temperature is fourteen degrees Fahrenheit. Blink a few times, then dash back upstairs to swap out the kicky capris you're wearing for lined tights and a fleece jacket. Ponder mittens but decide you don't want to carry them for most of the run, because you know you'll want to claw them off of your hands ten minutes in.

Lace up shoes and head outside. Feel the moisture in your skull freeze. Sigh heavily for a second or two. Shake unmittened fist at the low, gray sky. Then go.

Spend first mile remembering the mantra, "Never judge a run by the first mile." Because this first mile, like so many previous first miles, bites the big weenie. You think about a nice warm cup of coffee and a bowl of steel-cut oats drowning in maple syrup and butter. You obsess about the weird little ache in your right IT band and how it *has* to be the sign of something awful. And you know this running thing is a stupid way to start a morning when it is fourteen degrees outside and you are old and fat and slow.

But mostly you think about that oatmeal.

Around mile 3, you experience what you've been calling "the Dumbledore effect," after the scenes in the Harry Potter movies and books, where the wizard gathers up his memories with the tip of his wand and puts them in the Pensieve, which is the stone, birdbath-like dish where thoughts can be sorted and stored for later viewing. Running is your Pensieve, the place you can put all those mental cotton-candy wisps you accumulate over a day, a week, a life, so you can look at all of them objectively.

You Dumbledore your way through miles 4 and 5, too, sifting through various kid crises like your tween daughter's poor organization skills and your eight-year-old boy's addiction to video games. You wonder about your career, if you'll ever sell another book proposal or write anything worth keeping. You decide leaving the mittens at home was the right call while you unzip your jacket just a smidge because you are overly toasty. The fourteen-degree air feels delightful now.

You also worry about your aging parents, how far away each one lives, and wish you had a sibling who could take some of the load. You make a note to put gas in the car and, maybe, while you're out, get some ice cream. Or maybe those iced cookies you like from Panera.

You let a lot of it go because there's nothing concrete to be done about any of it, and it's hard to maintain that much angst when your legs have found a rhythm.

You pull out a gel from an outside pocket in your fleece jacket just before mile 5 and discover the cold has morphed its consistency to that of toothpaste. It's also your least favorite flavor: peanut butter. Slurp it down anyway because you could use the jolt. You move your emergency gel—the one you carry but don't think you'll need—to an inside pocket to warm it up a little, just in case.

Then it hits you that having a least favorite gel means you are a real runner.

After mile 5, you turn around, cross the street, and head back the way you came. You love to run an out-and-back because you can convince yourself it's not a 10-mile run, but, rather, a 5-mile run you do twice because you have to get home somehow. You've chosen this particular route carefully. The "out" is uphill, which makes you strong even as it ticks you off, especially the near-vertical incline at mile 4 that makes you want to vomit three-quarters of the way up. The "back" is blissfully downhill, which feels like flying when your legs are tired and always leads to negative splits. Both knowing the term *negative splits* and achieving that state makes you feel like a badass.

Because you live in a town where there are a surprising number of runners, you play the waving game, in which you wave at every passing runner, just to see who waves back. Women always do. So do men about your age. Young men never do, for reasons about which you can only speculate. It's hard to be young and male. Young men are told all that matters is being faster or stronger or richer than the guy next to you, which makes it so hard to focus on anything else like, say, that slow, old lady waving at you.

It's hard to be young and female, too, but for different reasons, like never feeling like you're pretty enough or kind enough or determined enough to be worthy of love. You wouldn't go back, even though you do miss your twenty-five-year-old hips and knees.

You could be wrong about all that, too. You've been wrong about a lot, frankly.

For instance, take how you thought you would never, ever be a runner. Through miles 7 and 8, you remember how freaking hard it was just to get through 1 mile only a couple of years ago. You were driven to run when a friend's snapshot showed you just how much weight you'd gained in your late thirties. You recall how five minutes of running was about all you could stand before you had to slow to a walk and how only thirty minutes of a run/walk cycle would leave you wrung out and breathless.

And, now, here you are, out on runs that span hours. Which doesn't mean they are easy. The size of the challenge is still just as enormous; the specifics of the challenge have mutated. You no longer worry if you can just keep your legs moving for a mile. Now the worries are about seeing how far you can go. Then, once you get a half-marathon under your belt, which is why you're out here in subfreezing weather on the first day of spring running 10 miles in the first place, you plan to see how fast you can go.

There's always something else to reach for, with running and so many parts of life. It's never easy, and the only answer seems to be persistence. Which is a lot of thinky thoughts, you think, for such a simple run.

Your Garmin bleeps to let you know you've started mile 9, which you convert in your head to a simple phrase: 1 mile. You try to forget the other nine you've just done and how nice it would be to just sit for a second. Those previous miles are in the past. Right now, you only have to run 1 mile. Just one.

You learned this during childbirth, this trick of forgetting the past contractions so you can focus on what's happening right now. It didn't work terribly well in the teeth of labor; it seems to work on the long runs, as long as you don't think too much.

Which is fairly easy by this last mile. Only two thoughts occupy your brain: This is how horses feel when they can see the barn, and, man, you really need to pee after being out in the cold for nearly two hours.

Then you are home. You grab a glass of chocolate milk on your way upstairs—climbing the stairs feels alien after running so long and your legs are confused—and bond with your foam roller before luxuriating in a nice, long shower.

Or that's the plan. What really happens is you roll out your quads while grousing at the children to do their dang chores and rush through your shower because you forgot the oldest one needed to be at the mall selling Girl Scout cookies about ten minutes ago.

For a brief moment, you wish you could put your running shoes back on and head out again.

Instead, you grab your car keys and go.

TAKE IT *From* A MOTHER
WHAT PARTS OF RUNNING GIVE YOU JOY?

"Running outside on a quiet street, having an awesome playlist, and singing along at the top of my lungs."

— LAURAL ("I sometimes throw my arms in the air, too, and I generally don't get caught, but one time an older gentleman started to sing along. It was fabulous.")

"Going farther or faster than I thought I could."

—ALICIA (After sprinting against a guy to a finish line, "he approached me afterward and said he was racing *me*. I was honored to keep up with him!")

"On a 3-mile loop close to my house, I always sprint the last corner home. Letting it all out makes me feel free."

—MERYL (Perfect running weather: fifty-five and sunny. Or seventy and rainy.)

"The end. I always tell people I don't enjoy running, but like having run."

—KAREN (Has been running for eight years, but still feels "like a newbie three out of five runs. The first 3 miles always suck. What is up with that?")

"Finding myself in the company of other ladies on a Sunday morning, all united in that morning's quest for a happy finish line."

—ANNE (Doesn't weigh herself, but went from a size sixteen to a "baggy eight" in the two years since she's been running.)

"Mile 7. I love mile 7. I've put some good time and distance behind me, and I feel like I can do anything."

—KRIS (Has an exceptionally supportive spouse, "but he isn't everything: I still have to drag my ass out of bed.")

"Trail running."

—EMILY (Her best running friend is Lindsay, whom she met working in the oil fields of Prudhoe Bay, Alaska, twenty years ago. "We walked then, patrolling for bears." They both now live in Portland, Oregon, and run together three days a week.)

"Cracking open a really cold beer after a run. It always tastes better then."

—TANA (Favorite training move: warrior progression in yoga. "Being able to hold a great plank is also empowering.")

"Races! There is something about seeing that finish line that makes me feel invincible. If there were no races, I'd be a lot less motivated to get in all the training runs."

—LAURA (Has run 79 races in the three-and-a-half years since her first 5K.)

"I love being outside on my own, listening to tunes. I love running with friends: a social outing with health benefits. I love reading about running, working on a training plan, and shopping for races."

—SUSAN ("Five years ago, if you'd have told me I'd say this, I would have laughed and thrown a french fry at you.")

"Feeling healthy—and looking better than I have in twenty-five years doesn't hurt either."

—GINA (Her goal is to volunteer at more races than she runs.)

"I love the feeling of pushing my body past the point where I think I can hang on without gasping or having to stop altogether. It's like a door opening before me, and I begin to settle in with extra oxygen and renewed strength in my legs."

—CINDY (When she climbs a hill, she leans forward, pulls in her core, and pretends little hands are holding and lifting her butt up the hill. "I know you are laughing, but try it next time and you won't think I'm so crazy.")

"Being alone. My solo runs are therapy for this introverted mama."

—CATHY (Loves listening to Macklemore. "Seriously, I owe my entire year of running to that man.")

"A good sweat. 12 x 400s is my favorite workout."

—ANNIKA (She's a homeschooling mom of five. "Running has counseled me through failed IVF, miscarriages, and two adoptions gone wrong.")

"The feeling I am now a runner, after being envious of runners for years."

—MAYA (Loves hill repeats. "Over fast, and they don't feel as hard as a sprint.")

A GHOST STORY

by Marit Fischer

I run with ghosts. Not all the time, just once in a while.

It all started with Amy. Amy was a friend of a friend who disappeared while running in the Wind River Mountains in the summer of 1997. I had never met her, but I recognized her name in a *Denver Post* headline one Sunday morning, and I read, without breathing, the story investigators and reporters were piecing together. I was immediately drawn into the community's unwavering effort to find her, and drove from Denver to Lander, Wyoming, to help with the recovery effort. The thought of her being taken and hurt, probably raped, maybe murdered, was devastating, and it was impossible for me to accept she had been plucked from her world while running alone in the mountains. As a trail runner, that scenario was the most horrifying thing I could imagine.

My runs became reconnaissance missions. I looked for Amy everywhere, even hundreds of miles from where she had last been. I looked for her alive. I looked for her body. I looked into the eyes of other runners I met on the trails for any sign they knew where she was. While searching for her, I made up countless dialogues between us in my mind. These imaginary conversations were all me. I read her lines, and I read mine.

One day, years later, that changed. I was running alone on an exposed ridge through one of those sunrises that dyes the world pink like an Easter-egg bath. I was thinking about nothing but that color. Suddenly, a voice that was not my own, that had to be hers, told me clearly that she was not coming back, that it was time for me to let go.

I realized then true answers to life's questions don't appear by desperately making up options in my own head. I had been cluttering my mind with wishful thinking and worst-case scenarios, and in the process, creating a multiple-choice test of possibilities without a single correct answer in the mix. When I finally shut up and just lost myself in the run, I got the answer I'd been looking for, and I got it directly from the source. In a wash of emotion, I was simultaneously relieved of my burden, and thrilled at what I might learn and experience in the future through the simple practice of open-minded running.

That was my first run with a ghost.

There's more to welcoming ghosts than just being open. In the years since my first ghost run, I've learned a few more things about how to do it. If you want to run with ghosts, you have to run alone. If you've got company, your ghosts are not going to interrupt. They only want to talk to you.

The distance of the run is irrelevant, and so is the tempo. It's all about the rhythm you create and fall into. The heartbeat and footfall of running both eases your mind and sends out the invitation. Also, you have to be in your element. I, personally, have to be on trails. I feel at home on the ones I've traced a hundred times, but I find the same sense of familiarity on new trails, too. Part of this is the calm I feel when I'm doing what I love; part of it is the ingrained muscle memory of moving myself up switchbacks and over rocks and fallen trees; and part of it is the collective subconscious of all trails everywhere. It's like they're all kin, and I'm a friend of the family.

It's not always easy on a run to achieve the open state of mind that allows ghosts to visit. Runs are a time to think of work, relationships, kids, what to make for dinner. Just like when you're running with company, ghosts won't interrupt when you're processing your day. Sometimes, ironically, distraction lies in the very activity that enables ghosts to come in the first place: running. Running is the invitation when you're feeling good and your movement is effortless, but sometimes running hurts. On those bad days, when it's hard and your body won't cooperate, your mind will most likely be transfixed on your physical self. It won't be open. If you can't transcend the distraction, there will be no ghosts.

Just to be clear: Running with ghosts is not a freaky, possession-type thing during which I run down the trail with my eyes rolled back in my head, mumbling holy gibberish from frothing lips. It's peaceful. I'm contemplative. And I look completely normal—or as completely normal as any endurance trail runner looks while in the act. The only evidence of ghosts is in my mind. They fill my head, and then I make sense of why they're there. It's a two-way deal, though. I'm running along, tuned into listening, ready to understand, and then they come.

Since Amy, most of my ghosts have been a whole lot less weighty. Grandma Florence, for example, in her monogrammed dresses and costume jewelry, was a senator's wife with strong opinions and an impenetrable deflector shield against casual chitchat. She thought I was the best thing since Tab and Oreos, though, and we were quite a pair. In the last few years of her life, there were several times she snapped out of her melodic state of delirium to share lucid, relevant insights about things in my life she should have had no idea about because I hadn't told her anything about them. She was so out of it the rest of the time that it would have been easy to dismiss this as crazy talk, but it wasn't. She was somehow connected to me.

These days, Grandma Florence comes around occasionally to let me know I've figured something out. I'll be running along contemplating a recent decision, and suddenly I'll hear her belting out: "Hello, Dolly! Well, hello, Dolly! It's so nice to have you back where you belong!" Grandma Florence, Louis Armstrong, and I used to sing her favorite song together in her living room, with

Louis in the form of black vinyl spinning on her 1960s cabinet turntable. When I hear her now, I know for certain that whatever it was I was doing wrong, I'm doing it right now.

Frank, though, is quiet. I don't hear my stepdad talking; I just sense him. Sometimes I see him, too, the way he was before cancer: all healthy and sun-brown, with curly grey hair spilling out under his fishing cap, wearing his I'm-so-proud-of-you grin. Before he died when I was sixteen, he taught me how to camp and how to cook; how to be tough and how to laugh at myself; how to tell stories and how to sit without talking for hours; how to drive a car and how to run softly on the earth with quiet feet. Frank, if only through his silent, peaceful presence, has a lot more to share with me that will help me buff my roughs and sharpen my dulls. I welcome him as long as he wants to come.

Today, as I set out on a familiar trail that climbs steeply into the Wasatch Mountains, I can't calm down. My breathing is labored. My legs ache. My mind is stuck on me and my weakness and my disappointment, and I can't set it free. I am preoccupied by my own obsessive negativity, so I try to think of Barney.

My husband's dad is not well. He has outlived his prognosis twice now and clings to life, thanks to seventy years of stubbornness. Cancer wants to claim its prize and is growing impatient, but Barney is not ready yet. He's getting weaker, though. Once a giant presence with wit like a whip and a wallop of a laugh, he is now wispy, whispery, and wilted. He hardly eats. He can take a few steps on a good day, but standing is often too much for him. He crumples back into his chair, broken and weeping, and desperately wanting this, all of this, to be different. And then we all go blind with tears and sit quietly, reassuring him with gentle hands, and desperately wanting this, all of this, to be different.

I gasp, so painfully aware that it will not be long before Barney can join me on these ghost runs on the trails if he wants to, free from his sick body and his frustration. And even though that relief would be so welcome, like him, I am not ready yet. Saying goodbye, even with the promise of a mountainside meet-up, is desperately hard.

I keep climbing, hiking now, then forcing myself to run again, trying to offer my pain to Barney because I know this is the kind he would prefer.

I push on and climb higher, passing two trails that would have taken me down, that would have given me easy outs back to the car without any more self-inflicted inconvenience. No thank you. Not today. I keep going. I know where to, and it is important I get there.

At the peak, the trail flattens out and winds at a gentle grade for about a half-mile through the just-new green grass and wildflowers. Through a patch of aspens, the trail forks. I go left, to Emily's place. My running partner and I stumbled upon this place two summers ago, but I have not yet been there alone. Right at the edge of some spindly scrub oaks, perched on a small rise overlooking the Wasatch Mountains to the south and west and Park City to the east, is a bench made from an old chairlift chair. Someone refitted it with fine wood for its back and a soft weatherproof cushion for its seat, then carried it up there and secured it to the top of the mountain. The bench is a memorial for a woman named Emily. I didn't know her before, but now Emily is one of my ghosts.

On a plate that runs across the top of the bench is a message that reads: "*It's the views, those little things. You know, the wonders of life. —Emily Roosevelt 1969-2010.*" The first time I read it and looked out from this place, I connected with Emily. Her message resonated in me like a voice in a canyon, bouncing off the walls of my body and filling me up.

I stand there today next to that bench, breathing hard and turning slowly, taking in my world. Then I cry. I cry because this is not a place to be taken for granted. I cry because I know how lucky I am. I cry because I am alive, and I am so grateful. And then, I say out loud, "Thank you."

I turn around on the trail, wipe away my tears, and run. I smile and run as fast as I can, down, down, down. With me come my ghosts: Grandma Florence and Frank and Amy and Emily, and Barney too, in spirit but not yet in a ghost's free form. And on that descent, as I collect wind in my hair and salt on my skin and dirt on my shoes, I decide when I die, I will come back and visit my loves on ghost runs, too.

I also decide I want to leave a place, like Emily's, for anyone who needs it, for my daughter, my friends, and for people I haven't yet met, as a reminder of the important things, the little things. The things only ghosts, sometimes, can teach.

CELEBRITY DREAM RUN

Sometimes, on runs, our brains wander to places they'd never go while we're standing still. Memories of our firstborn's first steps. The entire lyrics to "Firework." Schematics for a laundry-folding machine.

So we decided to take this power and assemble a dream team of mother runners: women who inspire us to try harder, run faster, dig deeper, but at the end of the day, are still wiping kids' noses, signing permission slips, and loading the dishwasher just like the rest of us. And then we decided we'd insert ourselves into the pack of them.

A few details about this dream run: We're running an easy, chat-able pace. "I don't even know what my pace is on an easy day, except it is slow enough to enjoy a fun conversation with my teammates," says Deena Kastor, American women's record holder in the marathon. Since Dimity and Sarah are among Deena's teammates today, we're holding steady at a nice 10-minute-per-mile trot. And since we can run anywhere in the world, we're putting in our miles on a route in Wellington, New Zealand, called Across the Tops. "After a 15-minute climb, you traverse across the tops of hills," explains running pioneer Kathrine Switzer about one of her favorite routes. "You see sheep in meadow, windmills in the distance, the city, the sea. You look over the world."

Oh, and while the run is totally imaginary, the words actually aren't: We interviewed all these amazing athletes.

THE DREAM RUNNING POSSE:

NAME	ATHLETIC RESUME	OFFSPRING	COOL TIDBIT
Magdalena (Magda) Lewy Boulet	2008 Olympian in marathon	1 son	Loves short, intense hill repeats. "You learn to hurt, a quality useful in distance running."
Shayne Culpepper	Two-time Olympian in 1,500- and 5,000-meters	4 sons	Was once surrounded by cows while running in an open space. "They're bigger up close than you'd think they'd be."
Jennie Finch	Two-time Olympian in softball and marathon finisher	2 sons + 1 daughter	Convinced her running group in Louisiana to try a triathlon.

NAME	ATHLETIC RESUME	OFFSPRING	COOL TIDBIT
Lauren Fleshman	Two-time 5,000-meter American champion	1 son	Favorite workout is a long run, followed by brunch with friends.
Kara Goucher	Two-time Olympian in 10,000 meters and marathon	1 son	Mantra: I am limitless. "There's no expiration date, no standards."
Deena Kastor	Two-time Olympian in marathon; holder of American marathon record	1 daughter	Loves the 18-mile Thousand Island Lakes loop in Mammoth, CA. "Most astonishing place I have seen in the entire world."
Roisin (Ro) McGettigan	Olympian in the steeple-chase	2 daughters	Three words that describe her current running: different perspective now.
Summer Sanders	Olympian in swimming and eight-time marathon finisher	1 son + 1 daughter	Dissects her goal for a race—go fast, come back from injury, enjoy time with friends—then sets her training plan accordingly.
Kathrine Switzer	First woman to run Boston Marathon with a numbered entry; winner of 1974 New York City Marathon	Millions, including you	After running Boston, she founded the Avon running circuit, which set the stage for the women's marathon to be included in the 1984 Olympics for the first time. "I'm 67, and still empowering women. I can't wait for what's next."
Carrie Tollefson	Olympian in the 1,500-meters	1 daughter + 1 son	"Growing up, I had the best runs with my Dad. Some of my favorite memories."
Christy Turlington Burns	Two-time marathon finisher; returned to running to raise funds and awareness after a potentially fatal labor and delivery	1 daughter + 1 son	Founder of Every Mother Counts, a non-profit that advocates for maternal health around the world. "Women around the world travel over 5K on foot to reach basic care; for emergency care, it's closer to a marathon."

DIMITY: "So we're all happily out here now, but first things first: Do you ever not want to run?"

LAUREN: "Yes! I'm tired! I'm a mom! A wife! I have a job!"

SHAYNE: "Yeah, for sure. And now when I don't want to run, I don't . . . unless it's been too many days in a row of not going."

MAGDA: "I just remind myself I always feel better after a run than I did before one. And once I get going, I hardly ever want to stop."

JENNIE: "I'm traveling a ton lately, and have three little ones who are my priority—along with getting sleep when I can. Those factors trump my runs. I'm hoping to get back into a better routine soon; in the meantime, I'm trying to be patient with myself. But I miss those runs!"

CARRIE: "All the time. I am busy, sore, and sometimes just bored with running after so many years. Sometimes, I have to just sit around the house for an hour or two with my running clothes on, and then, when I finally head out, go at an easy pace."

LAUREN: "I'm not a fashionista, but I believe in the power of a cute running outfit. Just like a power suit gets you in the state of mind for a presentation, a good workout outfit can prime your mind for a workout. It's science: *enclothed cognition.* Look it up!"

RO: "When I'm dragging, sometimes I just run to the top of my road and back. A 10- to 15-minute run gives me fresh air and changes my whole mood."

CARRIE: "So get that. I'm the master of the 20-minute run. It's not long, but it's better than nothing. I'm so happy I got out and always feel better after it."

SUMMER: "After having a kid, you've got to cut yourself some slack. I call it *momnesia:* You forget what your body has just gone through. You have to be smart, patient, and forgiving. Realizing you don't have go 110 percent all the time—and saying it out loud—is huge. The more I said it, the more it sunk in."

KARA: "My son does the verbalizing for me. I'm good with motivating for morning runs, but afternoon sessions are harder. The longer I wait to run, the worse it is. After a while, Colt, my son, will be like, 'Just go, Mom!'"

LAUREN: "Running buddies are key. The times I'm most likely to flake out are when I have nobody to meet for a run, so I schedule run dates as often as possible."

SARAH: "Right on, Lauren, I hear you there. I meet my pal Molly three mornings a week, and I look forward to seeing her every time. Who is your favorite running partner?"

CARRIE: "I love to go for a run with my husband. He's not much of a talker around the house, but get him on a run and ideas about our future and kids come pouring out."

SUMMER: "The moment my friend Kate and I push lock on our car keys, our conversation starts. Our feet start moving, the words keep flowing. She pushes me out of my comfort zone; we run on trails I wouldn't run alone and up hills I'd rather not climb."

KATHRINE: "I always tell women to find a good running friend, but I like to go with just the birdies above me. I'm constantly surrounded by people, which I love, but I need some alone time and space. Running gives me that."

KARA: "I go in waves between running solo and with training partners. It kind of correlates with how my life is going; when I'm going through a lot of stuff, I like to be alone. My life is pretty clean right now, and I'm enjoying company and chatter."

JENNIE: "When I was training for the New York City Marathon, a stray dog followed me for 10 miles. I convinced my husband we should keep him, and now he's our dog, named Bullet, and he runs with me. I always feel safe with him beside me."

DEENA: "I love running with my Mammoth Track Club teammates, but casual runs with my family are the best. One night last week, Andrew, my husband, pulled Piper, our daughter, in the bike trailer while I did a recovery run. Just after we started, she wanted to get out and run. We covered slightly more than a mile in 35 minutes, but seeing her experience such joy had me soaring."

DIMITY: "Thirty-five minutes at three years old: might be a world record. How often do you get asked if your kids will be runners?"

DEENA: "Every day! And she clearly *is* a runner—and she'll be whatever she wants to be with her attitude! After watching *Black Swan*, we agreed she can be anything except a ballerina, which is what she'll probably take to, of course."

LAUREN: "Since my husband is pro triathlete, people make jokes about our baby inheriting crazy athlete genes. I just smile. As we all know, it takes a hell of a lot more than genes to be a runner. It's a mindset, a lifestyle, and no amount of mitochondria or VO$_2$ max number can guarantee you'll enjoy the pursuit of running. Selfishly, I hope I can trail run with my son one day because I love him and I love running, but that's not up to me."

SHAYNE: "My boys are a little older, and my oldest is an avid tennis player. We made him run cross-country to get a little diversity in his athletics, and he won a countywide race without much training: He covered 1.5 miles in 9 minutes. But once you become a parent, you realize the choice is up to the child."

MAGDA: "I get that all the time, too. I usually just say he runs all over the place, which is true."

KARA: "When we bring Colt to races, he calls me 'Kara Goucher' instead of Mom. Totally cracks me up."

SARAH: "Nice segue for me, *Kara Goucher*. Racing: What's your favorite distance?

DEENA: "I love the half-marathon. It takes less out of me without cheating me out of the immense satisfaction of crossing the finish line."

JENNIE: "Me, too. I've run three halfs, and I'm able to pull them off without too much training. It's long enough to feel like you've put in some good distance and accomplished something big."

CHRISTY: "Another vote for 13.1. They require training and stamina, but, compared to marathons, I hobble around a lot less afterward."

RO: "I don't know if I'll get into the half-marathon buzz. I've been overtrained before, and that's the worst place to be: I was tired all the time, and have no desire to do that to myself again."

MAGDA: "My favorite distance is the one I have the most success at. It's changed over the years: I used to love the marathon, then the 5K for a while, and now I'm obsessed with 100-mile races, especially after pacing a friend at Western States."

KARA: "If I have to pick one, I'll go marathon. I love the training for it, and the race itself is so interesting: so many highs and lows. It's a thrill having people cheer for you for 26.2 miles. It's a high you don't experience anywhere else in running."

LAUREN: "You guys go long, I'll go 5K. You need endurance, speed, and strength for one, so there's a lot of variety to look forward to, and I feel like I'm becoming a better overall 'athlete' when I focus on it. I love competing on the highest stages around the world as a pro athlete, but I also love how easy it is to spontaneously jump in a 5K wherever I am."

SUMMER: "I have yet to figure out a 5K. I've never been able to sprint; it's just painful from beginning to end. I don't really have a favorite: I need consistent change. What keeps me fresh is a variety of races."

DIMITY: "Is there a particular race that stands out in your mind?"

SUMMER: "Definitely the 2014 Boston Marathon. After a red-eye from Hawaii, where we had an epic spring break trip with my husband's side of the family, we landed in Utah at 9 a.m., and I was on a 9:45 a.m. flight to Boston. I was exhausted and had an awful sore throat, and I was doubting my decision. I stepped on the plane, and there were so many runners and so much positive energy. They should've painted that plane blue and yellow. Having been at the 2013 marathon with the bombings, it was a therapeutic way to start the trip. I swear I had a fever on the bus ride to the start, but I took a couple of Advil—something I hardly ever do before a run—and set off. My long training runs were almost exclusively on rolling hills, like the Boston course, and they paid off. After mile 22, I had energy and legs to spare. It was just magical."

CARRIE: "Mine would be my first marathon, the Twin Cities. Crazy hard after having Everett, who was just four months and four days old—not that I'm counting or anything. It was so fun to be in my home state and surrounded by my family. I think I saw Jesus at mile 23. No joke: I was seeing all sorts of white clouds and envisioning the gates of heaven. I totally bonked and had to walk."

KARA: "I love racing in Minnesota, too. My prep race for the 2012 Olympics was in Duluth, my hometown; it was the USA Half-Marathon Championships. My grandparents, my high school coach, and so many other friends and family were there. It was the perfect send-off."

LAUREN: "I didn't make it to the London Olympics, but my proudest race moment was finishing last in the 2012 Olympic Trials after an IT band injury prevented me from training properly. There was pressure from the outside to bag the race from people who felt 'making the Olympic team' was the only goal that mattered, but it was important to find the courage to compete in the face of adversity, knowing I had no shot of making the team. I found the courage to set my own definition of success, and in the process I inspired a lot of people in unexpected ways."

JENNIE: "Way to turn a negative into a positive. I loved sprinting through the finish line of the New York City Marathon."

CHRISTY: "During one of my New York Marathons, I think I stopped to pee every mile from about mile 9 on. I was hydrating as I normally do, but my body could not retain the water. All that squatting was pretty tortuous after a while."

SARAH: "TMI! My favorite! Anybody else have a tough race moment?"

MAGDA: "That's an easy one for me. I injured my knee on the shuttle bus the day I arrived in Beijing for the 2008 Olympic Marathon. The swelling had decreased enough in the days leading up to the race that I thought I would be fine, but by halfway through the race, I couldn't put any weight on my knee. I had to stop."

RO: "Oh, those Olympics were tough for me, too. I was competing in the steeplechase, and had a really good semifinals. I was just floating through the course. The finals were the complete opposite:

My legs were not there. I couldn't jump over the hurdles. I fell in the water jumps. And the tough thing about steeplechase is you can't just jog it in: You still have to get over big obstacles. My heart was broken."

CARRIE: "Falling in a big race is no fun. I thought I was in the shape of my life for the World Cross Country Championships in 2006 in Japan. In the first 400 meters of the race, I fell down and lost all hopes of being in the top ten. Tough gulp to swallow."

KATHRINE: "In my thirty-nineth marathon in Athens, my quads seized around 30K, at nearly the exact point where Paula Radcliffe's legs gave out in the 2004 Olympic marathon and she sat down on the curb and cried. 'You poor woman,' I thought. 'I now know how you felt.' I somehow got to about 33K and Roger, my husband, came out on the course. I gave him hell, like it was his fault. He told me I could finish, and I said, 'I can't even walk. You have no idea.' He said, 'Okay, then stop and let's go home. You won't be the first person who quit a marathon.' I said, 'That's not an option,' and then hobbled off like Charlie Chaplin. The last 10K is downhill, and my muscles started to loosen. I burst into tears when I came into the stadium to finish. After the race, I apologized to Roger. It's crazy: I had my first moment of utter self-doubt at age sixty-five."

SUMMER: "I ran the Chicago Marathon in heat and humidity: my kryptonite. I thought I was at mile 22, when I was actually at 20. Mental blow right there. So I started thinking about something I read: Beginning runners focus on the pain; intermediate runners think about the distance; pro runners think about their form. I focused on my form, lifting my knees, relaxing my shoulders, concentrating on my breath. And I put a smile on my face. I really feel like if you display the pain you're feeling, it's going to be worse."

DIMITY: "That's a great philosophy: Smile to alleviate the pain. Was pregnancy painful for you—or was it more of a glowing time in your life?"

RO: "The first time I was in love with my body was when I was pregnant. Even though I was ripped when I was training for the Olympics, I didn't appreciate my body: It was always too this or too that. I loved my femininity and curves when I was pregnant. Maybe I was in la la land, but I was like, 'Forget this running crap. *This* is what my body is for.'"

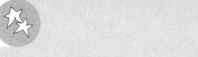

DEENA: "I couldn't run or exercise for the last five months of pregnancy without getting awful side stitches, so I lost a lot of muscle tone. I didn't panic, though; I knew I could rebuild myself after Piper was born."

CHRISTY: "In many ways, my body changed for the better after pregnancy. Before my first pregnancy, the only exercise I had done for many years was yoga, which taught me to accept and respect my body. After my second pregnancy, I started to crave more movement, so I started to incorporate more cardio like running."

LAUREN: "It took me quite a while to get my endurance back after pregnancy; my speed and power bounced back a lot faster. I was way stronger in the weight room from carrying all that extra weight around on my legs for months."

KARA: "I don't have my toothpick runner arms after having Colt. They're much stronger from carrying him around. My stomach isn't the same, either, but my long runs are so much stronger. I see the changes as a positive thing, not negative."

CARRIE: "So many changes after becoming a mom. I love running, but I've connected with people so much more now that I'm a mother runner. I gave my running career so much focus, I am fine with letting it be what it is now. I see no reason to miss a family meal or a swim lesson because I need to get in a run."

JENNIE: "Motherhood has made me more efficient in my workouts. If I'm going to be away from my kiddos, I better give it my all. Also, I know I'm a better mom when I'm an active mom. It's not just a physical thing—it's emotionally and mentally good, too."

SARAH: "You're a better mom when you're an active mom: Amen to that. But it begs the question: Which is harder, ladies: childbirth and/or mothering, or running?"

MAGDA: "Probably being a mother, but it's much more fulfilling than running could ever be."

SHAYNE: "Track intervals, but I was the type to get an epidural immediately."

CHRISTY: "Childbirth can be so challenging and marathon-like, but it is finite. I labored for twelve hours with my first child and four with my second. So I would say my first marathon and my second birth experience were pretty close—and that analogy made so much sense once I went 26.2. But mothering lasts a lifetime."

LAUREN: "They are totally different kinds of hard. As a mom, I can get help, share responsibility with my husband, enlist the help of grandmas and friends. That's not to say it isn't hard—because, holy moly, it's hard!—but it can be shared. To truly be your best in running, you can't outsource much, if anything. It's all on you. Even if you have a coach, nobody else can do your training. Nobody else can sleep for you. Nobody else can refuel. Nobody else can set your goals. Nobody else can run the race. This realization hit me just the other day as I was planning for the upcoming year and strategizing my support crew to help with the various parts of my life: motherhood, running, and Picky Bars. Running was the one where I went, 'Oh shit, that's all me.'"

DEENA: "Mothering! Marathons come with a concise training schedule and a finish line. Mothering, on the other hand, has no manual or end. I was prepared for lots of things about mothering—flushing dead fish down the toilet and tantrums—but I wasn't ready for Piper yelling things like, 'Start counting to three like you are going to put me in a time out and then I'll pick up the Play-Doh.' Seriously?"

KARA: "You have to just laugh, right? The other day, Colt was describing our family. 'Dad, you're the best. I'm the cutest,' he said. 'And Mom's a runner.'"

05

STRENGTH:
You Are More Badass
Than You Thought

"I will run in terrible weather. I will run
when I'm not feeling 100 percent. I will
run when I'd rather be sleeping. When I
get an opportunity to throw on my shoes
and head out the door, I will take it."

—SHANNON

I DREAMED WE WERE RUNNING

by Alison Overholt

I've never liked running.

In high school, I craved that instant *Yesssss!* that came with grabbing a rebound from right over someone's head in a basketball game, or the satisfaction of sprinting for a loose ball and knowing I'd beat the other girl as we scrambled down the court to get it.

By contrast, I *hated* those mile-run tests in gym class. And those "conditioning" runs our hoops team did semi-regularly after practice? *Kill me now.* That's what I thought every time we headed out. There was no sprinter's high waiting for me on the trail, just the feeling of legs turning to sandbags, breath ragged, with that near-instantaneous stitch in my side and blood thudding in my ears as I struggled not to fall too far behind.

The day I realized our coach didn't really pay attention once we headed out to run, and that, once out of his sight, I could detour off the park path to the nearby reservoir and leap off the bridge into the cool water below . . . well, that was possibly the best day of my senior year.

That's right. I literally jumped off a bridge just to avoid running.

Fast-forward twenty years, and I'm living in the 'burbs, working crazy hours, and there's not a whole lot of basketball happening in my life. Around here, women my age don't seem to have the time or interest in gathering for games, so I'm trying a spin class here, a yoga class there, but I'm mostly just cutting corners on the fitness front and starting to get used to the extra ten pounds I'm carrying.

Then, in early May of 2010, my mom got breast cancer.

And a month later, I got pregnant.

Sometimes I think of that summer as the one when someone pushed the "hyperdrive" and the "pause" button on my life exactly at the same time. All summer, I was back and forth between New York and Texas to help with doctors' appointments, paperwork, and postsurgical care, while furtively sitting in on conference calls from hospital waiting rooms, editing stories as my mother napped, answering e-mails on my phone in bathroom stalls.

Despite the frenzied activity, it also felt as if, for those few months, the world simply stopped spinning. (And not just when I took a "break" to puke in the bathroom, when pregnancy nausea got overwhelming.) It was as if everything got terribly quiet. I had this sense I was paying close attention to *life*, noticing every single detail I normally might blow right past: My mother's hand resting lightly on my arm as we watched the Red Sox on TV, her nails—always perfectly oval and impeccably polished —reflexively digging into my skin at every out. The sound of her too-loud telephone ring, as jarring as ever, but now a reassuring reminder of how many people cared enough to call at all hours of the day to check on us. The pulsing heat of each Texas summer day, which seemed to slow time—and everyone's speech—no matter how packed our days were.

Of course, there were some details I had always noticed. My entire life, I had watched my mother struggle with her weight, her confidence, and ultimately her health. She'd gain and lose the same fifty pounds over and over, dealing first with a thyroid issue, then high blood pressure, then diabetes, now cancer. My teenage self had always noted how angry she got when she struggled with clothes that had grown too tight—again—then judged her for not doing something about it. My adult self cried for her now, as she stood on the scale at the surgeon's office, making gallows jokes about how she could finally take off ten pounds when the doctors removed her breasts.

My mom died when I was five months pregnant. She and I both thought she'd beaten the cancer, and we were looking ahead to Thanksgiving, planning a weekend of crib shopping and celebratory feasting. But a week after her last chemo treatment, and the day after leaving me a raspy-voiced message where she whispered, "It hurts, Ali. The treatments are always hard, but it's really bad this time," she passed away from a pulmonary embolism. Her body just couldn't take it anymore.

The rest of my pregnancy still seems like some movie I watched at 3 a.m.; I know I was there, but the details are hazy, and there are bits I'm pretty sure I just skipped entirely. I recall a lot of snow that winter, a lot of phone calls about estate logistics, a lot of long hours at a job I couldn't quite remember why I was doing. Then a lot of her furniture and boxes arriving a couple of weeks before the baby was born, turning my house—and my life—into something that felt like it didn't quite belong to me anymore.

And then . . . joy. "The baby" was our daughter, Madeleine, and she was here, born the day after my mom's birthday. All the cliché things people said were true: After death, there was life. After the months of winter darkness, spring was here again, and with it, the light of this new life in the world. After all the crying—well, there was more crying. But these were the tears of a brand-new person, and also my own, as I recovered from delivering that new life, then tried to figure out how to breastfeed it. Maddie was this incredible presence, and I couldn't shake the superstitious feeling that some of my mom's huge personality had gone right into this tiny little girl.

I also couldn't stop thinking about how I wanted things to be different for her—and for me—than they'd been for my mom. I wanted to be healthy for her, to have energy to share all the adventures I wanted us to have together. In the first months after Maddie arrived, I worked hard to shed my baby weight and felt good when twenty-five pregnancy pounds disappeared, thanks to eating healthy and doing workout videos during her naps.

But I'd put on forty pounds, on top of the extra I'd already been carrying. And after that early weight-loss success, my efforts stalled. That hyperdrive button? Still in full effect. The plane trips and doctors' visits for my mom had simply given way to feedings and changings, mountains of laundry, and more doctors' visits—just different ones. Throw in my husband's travel schedule and my own work deadlines, and the feeling that life didn't quite belong to me was starting to feel permanent.

When Maddie was about eighteen months old, I stood in the kitchen holding my coffee in one hand and my own thyroid pill in the other, and thought: *This is how it happens.* Mom's struggle to "do something about it" didn't seem so simple anymore. I wished so much for just one moment, one chance to tell her I understood, now, how hard it was. I also thought about how I wanted to share something better with my daughter, to pass along more than a fraught medical history and a habit of avoiding mirrors.

So I started running. To clear my head. To get fit again. To just . . . do something about it.

Running was exactly as hard as I remembered from high school. My legs were the same bags of sand; my lungs still burned. But at 36, I'd experienced a lot of things in life that were so much more painful. This time around, the hardness of running seemed less of an actual obstacle, and more like a basic fact I acknowledged, then moved past.

The first day, I think I only ran for about 2 minutes before stopping to walk. But then I walked for a minute, and I started running again, and I did that for about half an hour. More importantly, I did it again the next day, and the day after that. And I did go a little bit farther each time I went out; eventually I was running for 4 minutes before I took my walk breaks. Whenever I wanted to quit, I'd imagine what it would feel like to see Maddie cheer for me as I crossed a finish line, and with that version of myself tucked in my head, I'd keep going.

After a month, I wasn't any faster, but I could tell I was stronger. So I continued running.

I remember the day I first made it 5 whole miles. It was a dull, gray winter day, and the thermometer on my car dashboard said sixteen degrees when I dropped Maddie off at day care. I went running anyway, wearing pretty much all my ski gear, from my long johns to my fleecy neck gaiter. All that was missing were my helmet and goggles. When my Garmin said I'd hit mile 5, just past the high school over on Park Street, I stopped and did an actual happy dance right outside the main building.

After reaching that milestone, it was like something inside me clicked; I just knew I was going to keep running. Some days I'd head out, singing along with my playlist, shutting out the world, and zoning in on the music for the entire run. Other days, after pushing past that first punishing mile, the music would fade to the back of my awareness, and I'd just see the road in front of me, or how sharp the outline of the leaves in the trees looked against the sky. I've written entire articles in my head on long runs, rolling words and phrases around in my mind as I alternate run-and-walk, four-and-one, then come home to bang it all out on the computer in one long whoosh. I've spent other runs gasping for air, tears streaming down my face, because that just happened to be the one time that week when I could stop checking off items on the endless list of our life, and finally just *feel* what I was feeling.

One foot in front of the other. Four-and-one minutes at a time. One mile and then the next. I followed that slow-and-steady plan all the way to finishing my first half-marathon, four months after I took my first step out the door. Five months later, I checked off another 13.1. And two months after that? The 2013 New York City Marathon, thank you very much—26.2 miles for the girl who used to jump off a bridge rather than go for a run.

The first mile still always burns and creaks and aches in a way that makes me roll my eyes like my sixteen-year-old self and think, *Seriously? Doesn't this part ever stop?* But somewhere just shy of the 2-mile mark, when my legs find their rhythm, and my breath evens out, and I swear I can see the world more sharply as the fog clears from my mind . . . that's when I discover, as I find I have to do every single time I hit the road, that while I will never *like* running, I have grown to love it. It's a love that connects me to my mom, connects me to *me*, and connects my mother to the grand-daughter she never met.

And it's a love that is creating a new and better legacy in my family.

My daughter, who is now nearly three, was wide awake, but still lying quietly in her bed when I went into her room this morning.

"Is it wake-up time?" Maddie asked.

"Yes. What are you thinking about?"

"Last night I was dreaming," she answered.

"What about?"

"I was dreaming about you. We were running."

TAKE IT *From* A MOTHER
HOW DO YOU KEEP NUMBERS—MILEAGE, FINISHING TIMES, AND THE LIKE—IN PERSPECTIVE?

"I don't really care about numbers. It's all social for me now."

—MELISSA (Had a near miss with a skunk she thought was an owl. "It was in a gutter, because at 5 a.m. in the dark, that's where owls hide, right?")

"Part of why it took me so long to start running is because I hate treadmills, and I was too embarrassed to run outside. Now that I'm coming back from injury, I'm just so damned happy to run I don't even think about comparing myself to others."

—KAREN (Her secret weapon is listening to P!nk. "She busts ass so hard on her music, I owe it to her to run.")

"I've resisted getting a GPS for a long time. I was afraid it would steal my joy of running and make me too competitive. I finally got one for Christmas, and I'm hoping it wasn't a mistake."

—STEPHANIE (Her husband often pushes her out the door. "I hope because he knows I need it and love it, not because he wants me gone.")

"I struggle with comparing myself to others in so many ways. One day I decided instead of feeling badly about myself for my weaknesses, I'd let people know when I recognized a strength in them that I envied. It evolved into having a lot of great conversations about how we are often too hard on ourselves."

—KEIGHTY (Started running when she was fourteen. "I just put on my tennis shoes and went out the door, running all the streets in my neighborhood, jamming to an 'N Sync CD.")

"As long as I know I put my best effort out there, I'm good."

—MARY (Favorite prerace dinner is a burger with fries and a beer.)

"I only compare myself with myself. I could care less what pace others are running, but I love beating my own times."

—DIANA (Treat after a long run: rest!)

"One of the advantages of having started to run at age fifty-five is I don't have to compare myself to the young and the strong. Well, some of the times posed by women my age are pretty scary, but I don't have anything to prove anymore. It's just me and my running shoes—and that cute skirt with the pleat at the back. . . ."

—NANCY (One of her mantras: "The car is a long way from here.")

"Not there yet. I compare myself all of the time to other runners. I need to focus on how strong I am and not how fast. It's hard. I'm a work in progress."

—MARIE (Favorite strength training moves are lunges and squats with a kettlebell.)

"I am the queen of spin: I usually manage to convince myself slow numbers were due to some sort of external factor like weather."

—AMY (Doesn't have an official running streak, but hasn't gone more than one day between runs unless there was a medical reason.)

"Because I'm a decent local runner, other people are constantly pointing out other women I'm competing against. I hate competing. I have to tell myself over and over, 'Run your own race. Your best is enough.' It's a constant struggle, especially when everybody around me is doing the comparing for me."

—KIMBERLY (Spent a season *not* racing locally so she could run anonymously.)

"I convinced a friend to start running, and it seems easy for her. This I don't mind. But her race pictures are fantastic and mine always look spastic. That would really piss me off if she wasn't so nice."

—JANA (Not sure her mother "gets" her running, "but after years of seeing me get beat up in the martial arts, she doesn't say much.")

THE MIDDLE FINGER
by Susan Schorn

One Saturday afternoon each month, I untie my black belt, take off the white karate uniform I wear when I train at my dojo, and don street clothes to teach a women's self-defense class. All kinds of women attend these classes: old and young, tall and short, quiet and talkative. My goal is to teach them basic safety strategies, but also—more importantly—to help them become aware of their own capacity for power. I want them to feel their strength and how it can make them safer. During each three-hour class, I help them learn to use their voices, set boundaries, and defend themselves physically. Yet we spend the most time talking about running. As I have discovered, running lies at the heart of successful, empowering self-defense.

To help my students see how running can keep them safe and strong, I teach them a mnemonic device called "The Five Fingers of Self-Defense." Together, my students and I count off five important self-defense strategies on our fingers: *Think. Yell. Run. Fight. Tell.* Each word encompasses a spectrum of responses from the immediate level (*think* of an escape route) to big-picture applications (*fight* for policies that reduce systemic violence).

"The first finger," I explain, holding up my pinkie, "is *think*. It covers all the ways we can use our minds to reduce risks: Seeking out good information. Believing we are worth defending."

"*Yell*"—I hold up my ring finger—"refers to all the ways communication can help us stay safe. Saying, 'You're standing too close. Back off.' Or, 'I don't answer those kinds of questions.'"

"*Run* is the middle finger, and I won't show that to you by itself." This always gets a laugh. "But I love the fact that *run* is the middle finger because I believe it's the most powerful way to respond when someone threatens my safety. There's no more powerful way to defy violence than to simply not be there for it."

"*Fight*"—my index finger—"is pretty self-explanatory, and my thumb represents '*tell*,' which is an important part of safety because silence is one way survivors of violence are prevented from healing."

"Each of the five fingers represents a valid way to defend ourselves," I tell the students. Then I make a fist. "But we're safest when we use all five together."

That's the truth, but I have to admit: *Run* is my favorite finger.

I started running about a year after my son was born, when I was trying to work off the last five or ten pounds of pregnancy weight and, frankly, to get out of the house. I'm forty-six now, I have a daughter and a son, and I typically run anywhere from 6 to 20 miles a week, in addition to my martial-arts training. These days, I'm a solid mid-pack runner, whether I'm running a 5K or a half-marathon. I like longer distances but don't often have enough time to prepare for them. I no longer worry too much about improving my times. For me, running is primarily a way to hone my self-defense skills and keep up my cardiovascular strength.

In the evening, when I walk out my front door in south Austin to run, I'm not focused on the obvious self-defense applications of running: escaping from an attacker, for instance, or a more subtle use, such as getting off an elevator because of a creepy passenger. I'm not thinking in terms of physical escape at all, unless you count my desire to distance myself from the One Direction CD my ten-year-old daughter is listening to while she does her homework. As I start down my driveway, I'm just looking forward to the run, to all the things running gives me.

As I trot away from my house, I'm leaving behind my family: my daughter's habit of yelling at her math textbook, my never-ending cascade of e-mail, the half-prepared casserole my husband will have to finish and serve for dinner. Every step away from my household at this busy time of the day is a leap of faith that the world can muddle along without me for an hour or so, and that when I come back to it, I'll be able to handle any problems that might have arisen in my absence. By voluntarily giving up that kind of control, even for a short while, I have time to remember the only thing I am fully in charge of: myself.

My first rule of running is I always start downhill. This makes detaching from my family just a tiny bit easier: I'm not fighting guilt and gravity at the same time. As I ease down the gentle hill to the first turn on my route, I can feel the distance stretching out behind me, and it reminds me of other ways distance gives me power. Cutting off a disrespectful conversation. Leaving an unhealthy relationship. Telling a friend, "Thanks, but I need some space right now." All productive responses to situations that threaten boundaries and safety—and all slightly different ways of employing the strategy *run*.

Two turns into my usual 3-mile route to the railroad tracks and back, I start climbing, which gives me time to dig deeper into the meaning of *run*. (This is also part of my running strategy: If I don't occupy my mind on hills, I tend to hyperventilate.) As I bite into the hill, driving from the hip and staying tall, I realize runners have a much better intuitive understanding of distance—and the power it represents—than the average person. Runners know purposefully moving with our own energy takes us places, both physically and mentally, that we can't reach any other way. We know by transporting ourselves from one spot in the world to another, we change not only our location, but also our attitudes, our bodies, and perhaps our future. This is the essence of empowerment: not just reaching a new and better place, but *getting there on your own,* like to the top of this hill. Politicians and pundits talk about empowering women, but when you run, you *feel* it.

When my breathing has recovered from the hills, I usually get a fresh surge of energy, another reminder of why running is my favorite self-defense strategy. The sense of strength and freedom running generates—feelings that keep us running even when we're exhausted or bored or frustrated—can change lives. In self-defense classes, I teach women different ways to tap into personal power, but running gives me instant access to it. Every time I step out my door in my New Balance shoes, I turn into an amalgamation of Wonder Woman, Eleanor Roosevelt, and Tina Turner. This world often minimizes and dismisses women's autonomy, but each mile we run teaches us a lesson we can all stand to learn over and over again: I am powerful. I am strong. I control my own destiny. I can take care of myself. With each footfall, we reinforce these much-needed messages—and we're giving the figurative finger to everyone who believes otherwise.

Continuing down one long residential street, then another, I wave at some kids who go to school with my daughter. *They've already finished their homework*, I note silently. *They probably aren't allowed to listen to One Direction while they work.* I say hello to the retired couple who sits out on their porch swing every evening. The husband smokes a pipe, and the smell of tobacco always reminds me of my own father. I have time to contemplate the new free-form sculpture one neighbor has installed on his lawn. *Is it giant bird? A dinosaur? An abstract expression of despair?* (My neighborhood is usually accurately described by real-estate agents as "quirky.") Feeling at home on a street that isn't mine, I'm reminded of how running, an exercise in self-sufficiency, connects us to the larger world.

Racking up miles day after day brings us into contact with new people, and gives us fresh perspectives on places. I'm regularly struck by how different a street feels when I'm running on it instead of driving it. In a car, everything feels remote, as if I'm observing it through the glass of a museum display. Running, I feel the hardness of the pavement beating up through my feet with each step. I can hear and smell and sense every element of my environment: The game of basketball being played half a block away. The smoke from a backyard barbecue. I'm more aware of the people with whom I share the environment.

Practically everyone in my neighborhood knows I run. If they haven't seen me for a week or two, they'll ask where I was. They're not trying to make me feel bad for slacking off; they just want to know if I've been okay. This interest, I've discovered, is a great motivator. It reminds me my routine is important, even to other people. And it also makes me appreciate the role my neighbors play in making my community a safe place to live.

When we discuss the concept of *running* in self-defense classes, I ask students, "Where are the safe places in your life? Who are the people you would go to if you needed help?" On a practical level, this might mean knowing the name and phone number of your local police liaison. It might mean mapping out the restaurants and gas stations that are open for business when you do your regular predawn run. It can also mean having people who know you, and know your routines, and notice if something disrupts them. By running in my neighborhood, I've woven this additional layer of awareness surrounding me, a safety net the follows me wherever I go.

Self-defense skills continue to pulse through my run. As I navigate the loop by the railroad tracks, I *think* about crime reports I've seen for the area, and I keep my eyes and ears attuned for anything out of the ordinary. "Go ahead!" I call to the driver at the hazardous five-way intersection, using *yell* to avoid an accident. But as I pass the house with the goats in the backyard (like I said: quirky neighborhood) and turn for home, *run* again becomes the concept at the front of my mind.

Running isn't just about putting distance between us and the day, us and a problem, us and an unhealthy lifestyle. The motion also begs us to ask ourselves, *What are you running toward?* What do we want to move closer to? What are our goals? Once we appreciate our ability to move capably and confidently with our own power, it's important to ask, *Where are you going?* Because if we only go where we're told to go, where we're allowed to go, or where we're expected to go, we aren't reaching our full potential.

That's what I'm reminded of each time I run—and each time I count off the third finger of self-defense in front of a new class of students. In countless ways, running saves lives.

But more important, it gives us the kind of life that's worth living.

TAKE IT *From* A MOTHER
WHAT'S THE HARDEST YOU'VE PUSHED YOURSELF IN A RACE?

"The half after my mom died. I completely fell off the training wagon and almost bailed on the race. I went anyway, and put it all on the course: months of pain and sorrow. The last tenth of a mile was nothing but tears."

—TRACY (Ran 1:55 in that race, a PR by 15 minutes.)

"I ran a flat course for a 10K, and I really wanted to take several minutes off my PR time. I did it, but for once, when I finished, I had no kick at the end. There was nothing left."

—MELISSA (Weighed 300 pounds when she started running; she's since lost eighty pounds and runs three to six days a week.)

"Just recently I did my first 5K post-baby. I pushed so hard to break the 30-minute mark and finished in 29 something."

—MARIA (Pre-running, "I hated to sweat, and didn't like veggies and salads.")

"The weeks leading up to my first post-kid half-marathon, we went through three rounds of flu in our house; I was either sick or taking care of a sick child. It ended up being my slowest race ever, yet I never worked so hard to run so slowly. I left everything on that course, and it felt great."

—ZITA (Spoken like a true mother runner: "Pre-kids, I could barely make it to an 8 a.m. group run. Now I'm done with weekend long runs before eight o'clock.")

"Definitely the Chicago Marathon. I seriously remember about two minutes of the actual race. The rest of it is a blur of me trying to convince myself to keep moving and (successfully) trying to repress vomit."

—MARY JO (Complaint about running: "If I do it too much, my body hates me. If I don't do enough of it, my mind hates me.")

"This is actually something I'm trying to work on; I tend not to push myself. When I ran the Disneyland Half-Marathon, I wasn't even breathing hard until mile 12, which tells me I could try harder. But I'm afraid of burning out and not being able to finish."

—DIANE (When certain pieces of her running gear "won't de-stink," she soaks them in a tub of half water, half white vinegar before washing. "That always works.")

"The final mile of the Pittsburgh Half was a hill, where a woman was holding a sign that read, THIS HILL IS YOUR BITCH. *That sign gave me the attitude shift I needed in order to get up the hill and finish out the race on a high note."*

—LISA (Loves that race. "What a beautiful city, and those people know how to cheer!")

"My first full. There was a half going on at the same time, and it took every ounce of courage and strength I had not to follow the half course when it split. I doubted I could finish. Mile 17, I was hurting and wanted to give up. But by mile 18, I was feeling better, and there was great crowd support. I never got back to my five-hour finish, but I refused to let the 5:30 pacer catch up to me."

—NICOLE (Finished "with everything I had in 5:23:10. Best feeling ever!")

"I really pushed myself in a 5K in a forest preserve where a multiteam cross-country meet was going on. I was inspired by seeing all those hardworking, high school kids. I remember telling myself just to leave it all out on the trail. It felt glorious."

—MICHELLE (Made herself a rum and Coke after her first run and wondered, "Why do people choose to run?")

"During my first half-marathon, Boston's Run to Remember, I pushed so hard I had diarrhea and was vomiting during a postrace cookout we were hosting for Memorial Day. Awesome."

—KRISTIN (Sometimes her period makes her run faster. "Weird.")

UP THE DOWN ESCALATOR
by Michelle Theall

I am running, fast and furious, without thought to pace or form. Dirt from the Grand Canyon covers me with a red film kicked up from my shoes. My lungs burn, but I can't stop. I pass tourists strolling down the trail; they stare at me as if I am crazy. I pound my way down three thousand feet and 5 miles, leaving my family above me to wait and worry. I know I will be late—am already late—for the time we all agreed to meet back at the visitors' center. But momentum is all I have, and I'm clinging to it.

What if the next time I am here, I'm in a wheelchair?

I see the end of the trail. Another thought buoys me. *If I can do this, I must not be sick.* I reach the base and rest my body on a two-by-four post holding a temperature gauge. I blink twice. It reads a blistering 115 degrees Fahrenheit. My panting slows, and I grip my knees. *What am I doing?* Six months before, I would never have thought to take on the Grand Canyon in that kind of heat, without water and a clear plan articulated to others, but things are different now.

I glance around. The view up top where I've left people who love me was so much better than where I stand now. The steep walls seem to close in on me—and reality catches up to me. First, I still have to go back up this canyon. And second, I can't outrun my diagnosis of multiple sclerosis.

I've been a runner almost all my life, and throughout those forty-seven years, I've equated running with survival. I started running at age eleven, pigtails flying, after I was abused by a neighbor, then shortly afterward, by my best friend's father. I was too afraid to tell anyone what happened. Instead, I ran. By pumping my arms and sprinting through pain, I gained control of my world again. I felt strong enough to carry my secrets.

But running also became an obsession. I counted my teen years by the number of winged track patches on my letter jacket rather than the number of boyfriends or dances I attended. I studied the *Runner's World* annual shoe review the way other girls gleaned makeup tips from *Seventeen* or chose dresses for the prom. My parents, both former teachers, begged me to quit. Mom declared my ovaries would fall out and I'd be unable to bear children; Dad believed sports to be a cancer to the educational health of our country. "All that emphasis, glory, and money funneled toward a kid who can catch a football," he argued, "should be put toward math, reading, and science." I took home economics to appease my mother, and I kept my grades up. Still, I ran.

In 1985, after putting myself through two-a-day workouts, I landed a partial scholarship to run track at Texas Tech University. I competed in the 400 and 800 meters, and though I graduated summa cum laude, I didn't frame my diploma. Instead, I hung my old track spikes in my office at the athletic-shoe company where I landed a job after graduation. Despite my parents adamantly thinking otherwise, my running led me to the starting line of a career in sports that would span more than two decades and lead me to launch *Women's Adventure,* an active-women's magazine I developed for women seeking to live life to the fullest through outdoor sports, nature, and travel.

In 2002, while putting together the first issue of the magazine, I noticed a buzzing in my body. My coordination wavered. I knocked over drinking glasses and chipped plates. While running, I tripped over invisible objects, twisting ankles and sliding down scree. My fingers grew numb. My friends started warning me about curbs and stairs. My doctor ordered tests because, as a thirty-six-year-old female, I was a prime candidate for multiple sclerosis (MS). My MRI scans showed six white spots on my brain. A spinal tap confirmed the diagnosis. As the first issue of *Women's Adventure* hit the press in March 2003, my doctor called to tell me I had MS.

MS is a progressive, autoimmune disease with no cure. It attacks the central nervous system—the brain and spinal cord—causing scars that disrupt the path of neurological signals. Depending on the severity of the attack, its location, and the resulting scarring, the disease can leave a person temporarily or permanently paralyzed, numb, or blind. It can affect anything the central nervous system controls, which includes memory, bowel and bladder function, coordination and balance, sensory integration, swallowing. The only thing predictable about MS is its unpredictability. Everyone's path with MS is unique—and no one could tell me how quickly mine would travel.

After the diagnosis, I immediately attributed to MS every twinge, tingle, and tired muscle. I obsessed over my health, fearing the things I most loved to do might be stripped away from me. I lived to run, rock climb, snowboard, and backpack. To me, the most beautiful places were also the most remote. In 1997, I'd built my home in Colorado on ten acres with hiking trails, Continental Divide mountain views, and elk migrating through my land. I sought out quiet places, which were not along roadsides. They did not have wheelchair ramps. After trying one of the approved drugs to slow the progression of my disease—and having strokes in my eyes from it—I stopped treatment. My symptoms were irritating, but not debilitating.

On the one-year anniversary of my diagnosis—six months after I went down and up the Grand Canyon—I took stock of my health. My quads burned with fatigue, causing me to rest on landings between flights of stairs. Holding a cup of coffee taxed my reserves. The buzzing in my body escalated into twitching and involuntary movement. I began to punch and kick myself in my sleep. My magazine ran on autopilot, thanks to a dedicated staff that cut me a lot of slack while I tried to come to grips with my illness. My investor noticed my absence, but remained patient. And through it all, I thought about running.

Running had been my elixir, therapist, and cure for depression. Now, it became the barometer for how quickly my disease was progressing. In 2003, pre-MS, I could run 10 miles. A year later, a trip around the block seemed like a marathon. Did I still have any control? Had I tried everything in my power to regain my health? A little voice inside my head grew louder every day. It said, *You are giving up. Approach this like an athlete. Push through the hurt.* I was giving up things I loved without a fight. I decided to start training for my race with MS.

I created my own tough love, a thirty-day program. While I had never had a weight problem, I'd gained a good twenty pounds since college. My fatigued muscles deserved to be treated fairly; I had to stop asking them to carry extra weight. I identified my top two food vices—chocolate and alcohol—and allowed myself to eat chocolate on Wednesdays and drink alcohol on Saturdays.

Next, I researched supplements that would ease my muscle soreness, lessen muscle fatigue, and allow my mind and body to work together. Potassium, magnesium, calcium, B-12, B-100 complex, alpha lipioc, omega-3, and CoQ10 became part of my daily regimen. For my sticky muscles, which refused to glide over one another, I began getting a weekly myofascial massage to keep them fluid.

I started lifting weights and trying to run again. I reasoned that whatever signals could get through the scarred lesions in my brain to my nerves and muscles should be encouraged. Signals getting sent meant strength; blocked signals equaled atrophy. If I could walk a mile today, I could grocery shop in five years. If I could run a mile tomorrow, I could easily navigate international airports in ten years.

Making myself walk, then run, even when my body felt like a stiff paper clip being bent every which way, hurt my pride and my psyche. Running had been as effortless as breathing, and now it required conscious attention to every movement—otherwise I risked falling over. I tried to push away the big "what if": *What if I couldn't make it better?* I put one foot in front of the other, and one miraculous day in June, it got easier. Muscles glided over one another without unending spasms or cramping. Intense activity no longer ended up with me bedridden for days with fatigue and tremors. I recovered quicker, both mentally and physically, which allowed me to go farther and faster.

Six months later, I'd lost the post-collegiate twenty pounds and progressed to running 5 miles. I caught glimpses of the athlete I had once been, on the balls of my feet, arms and legs pumping. I changed from asking God for my health back, to thanking Him for returning it to me. I hesitated for only a moment when Mark, my best friend, called to say he was booking a group trip to Africa that would start with climbing Kilimanjaro and finish with a photo safari. I said yes, I would go, and started to dream of beasts howling in the dark and monkeys chanting. We would leave in September, just weeks away, and I resolved not to be the weakest link on our team.

There were days I wanted a banner on my chest that read: "Look what I can do. And I have MS." Those were the good days, when I was sprinting up a hill or rock-climbing an overhanging crag. Other days, like on the airplane to Africa, when I saw someone struggling to put a bag in the overhead bin, I wanted people to know there was a reason I didn't jump up to help. That although I looked young and healthy, I had a disease that on bad days left my arms so tired that petting my dog or stirring soup was tough.

Kilimanjaro rises 19,340 feet above sea level. Our forty-two-mile journey began at 8,692 feet. Practice hikes in Colorado, where I started at nine thousand feet and ended at fourteen thousand, gave me some confidence. Still, I didn't know what effect the thin African air would have on my scarred brain. On day two of the trip, I began to shake uncontrollably. My head bobbed, and my hands trembled. I joked I felt like Katharine Hepburn in *On Golden Pond.* "The loons, Norman. The loons!" Nervous laughter followed. I tried not to cry, but I was scared. *What if this was a bad idea? What if the shaking won't stop?* Mark grabbed my daypack. He wouldn't accept no for an answer. He clipped my pack onto his own and started walking.

At fifteen thousand feet, I grew nauseous, and my head filled with a dull ache that made me close my eyes. The pressure reminded me of the spinal tap doctors used to diagnose my MS—a test I swore I would never repeat. *Why exactly am I doing this?* I questioned my sanity for the first time in months and questioned our guide about alternative routes. He smiled. The only way to get to our path down was to keep going up.

At the final camp before our summit attempt, altitude sickness flattened me again. I skipped an acclimatization hike. My arms were so weak I could no longer hold my water bottle to drink, or even zip up our tent. I rested them in between attempts to grasp and yank at the zipper pull and Velcro. I remembered the Grand Canyon, now two years in my rearview mirror. It wasn't in my nature to give up, particularly where adventures were concerned.

But I listened to my body. And when most of our group left for the summit bid, I stayed behind. I wasn't alone. Jill, the woman I'd been in a relationship with for more than eight years, stayed with me. In the tent, our billowing temporary refuge of orange nylon perched above the clouds and strewn with water-purification tablets and wet wipes, we talked about adopting kids.

At the base of Kili, we'd watched children, who should have been in school, taking care of younger siblings; they were covered in dirt, holes in their clothes, besieged by flies. When we returned home, we decided we would start our family.

Eighteen months later, Jill and I adopted a thirteen-month-old boy, Connor, from foster care. Running after him has helped me put things into perspective. Pre-MS, I feared motherhood would hold back my running, a selfish activity that shouldn't take priority over a child who needed me 24/7. Now I see it the opposite way. I must stay healthy because of my commitment to him. Putting Connor in a jogging stroller adds an extra layer to my runs, along with laughter. We pet dogs and stop at playgrounds and hit the farmers' market. I tune into the world around me. I see it the way Connor does, with new vision and possibility.

I've lived with MS for more than ten years now. My runs are sometimes walks. But my walks sometimes become runs. Though there's not anything wrong with being a walker, I'm definitely not ready to label myself like that yet. I'm still a runner, and I continue to move forward, as fast as I can, with MS.

IN HER SHOES

Not sure about you, but neither Sarah nor Dimity will ever enter a 5K where everybody runs buck naked, minus shoes and socks. We'll never, ever win a marathon; watch a son with cerebral palsy cross a finish line; run a mile in less than five minutes; or pee during a race, no porta-potty required, either. (Okay, Sarah did that; Dimity never will.)

But that doesn't mean we're not curious about what it feels like to experience those feats, so this section is devoted to some good vicarious miles. (Just make sure another mother runner isn't right behind you if you're inspired to let it fly on the fly, like Sarah did.)

IN HER SHOES: LETTING IT ALL HANG OUT

I didn't know what my boobs were going to feel like when running without a bra. A week out from my first naked 5K, I did a trial run on my treadmill in the basement. I realized if the bouncing started to bother me, I could make little T-rex arms. That would hold them up. I also wasn't sure how chafed my big thighs would get.

Otherwise, running naked didn't seem so bad.

When my husband, a friend of mine from high school, and I drive through the gates of Sunny Rest Resort in Palmerton, Pennsylvania, to the Wiggle, Jiggle, and Giggle 5K, we immediately see our first penis. It's like: "Oh my God. There are balls. Holy cow. I can't believe it. Right there." The next thing we see is another guy, just walking his dog. Naked. Then some guy grilling. Naked. Which is a little scary to me. Not that he's naked—but that he's naked and grilling. Talk about a weenie roast.

We park the car. Then tackle a big decision: Do we strip in the car or do we get out and take our clothes off? We decide to strip inside, then climb out. For the first five seconds, it's unnerving because I'm just not used to being that naked, like, next to another car full of people who are also getting out naked.

Then I say to myself, "All right. I'm going to do it." I put sunscreen and Body Glide all over the place, and keep on my funky socks and shoes.

We walk up to the registration table. A lot of people at the registration table are naked. We check in. They write my number on my leg. As we wait for the start, people around us are stretching. Big guys sitting on the ground doing the hurdler's stretch with one knee back. Really just too much information there.

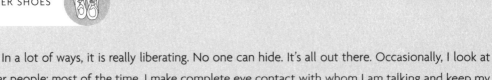

In a lot of ways, it is really liberating. No one can hide. It's all out there. Occasionally, I look at other people; most of the time, I make complete eye contact with whom I am talking and keep my focus above neck level. Every now and again, I see random awful C-section scars and lots of cellulite and lots of people who look pretty much like myself. That is really nice.

We line up like you do at any other race. There are maybe about 140 people. By the way, the nudists have no tan lines. Also, a couple of people—mostly women in their mid-thirties and younger—have clothing on. I think the clothed ones would probably be the best-looking ones naked. But I remember when I was in my twenties and thirties, I probably would not have been able to do it either.

The race starts. I hear a lot of giggling. I don't hear much flapping; I'd expected a lot more. I see a lot of well-groomed people. I don't see a lot of '70s bush. Everybody is very well 'scaped, which is interesting because I hadn't really given it much forethought.

We run on a road, past all of the RVs, where naked people are out having their coffee. They cheer everybody on. Then we run through woods and trails. The silence is beautiful.

We finish and have Gatorade and a banana. I stand around naked talking to other people. I don't mind it. At this point I've been naked for a good hour plus.

I put my clothes back on before the awards ceremony. It feels good to be dressed, but it's also a little bit sad because this experience is now over. I liked making myself a little bit uncomfortable; as a mom I've ratcheted down my level of crazy. Getting out there and taking a calculated risk was a freaking hoot.

I take sixth place in my age group, which is funny because it's the only running award I've ever received. Also, the age group was 40–59 and there might have been, like, seven people in the age group.

Still, that award is my claim to fame, and it sits on our mantle.

—PATTI (Ran the Bouncing Buns 5K the following summer.)

IN HER SHOES: MAKING MONEY ON THE MILES

I found a $20 bill in a puddle in the street one December morning. A mile later, I found a credit card. I rang doorbells to find the owner of the credit card, but I didn't ring any doorbells about the $20. (Side note: What does that say about my integrity?)

I told my girlfriend, a solo runner, about my two finds. We came up with the idea of collecting all of the change we each find over the year to see how much it would add up to. My goal was to get enough to buy a gel. Surely, I thought, I can find enough pennies to do that.

I don't find much in my neighborhood, but I live close to a major highway intersection and here in Texas we have frontage roads, which parallel interstates. I find a lot of change near stoplights on the frontage road. I think people here are just crazy and they dump their change out the window when they stop for the light. I have also started planning my routes the night before.

The most I have found in one run is $56. I was running along a frontage road at 6 a.m. on a Sunday. There wasn't any traffic. The money was in a washout from an elevated parking lot. I found a $20 bill. I picked it up, took a few steps, and—oh, my gosh—there's another one! And there's $10! And $5! I was so excited, I even took photos.

On another run, I found what I called a "pimp ring." It was gigantic. The sun in a parking lot hit it just right and the sparkle caught my eye. I took it to a jewelry store and got $240 for the gold (the stone was worthless).

I have a special jar for the run money. Although my husband contributes to it, too, he runs either at night or earlier in the morning when it's darker so he doesn't find as much. Plus, I don't think he has patience for it. He's much more focused on pace and time. He can't stop for that penny. I'm more than okay with stopping.

The most we've found in one year was just over $400. We donate the money to the Achon Uganda Children's Fund: Julius Achon is an Olympic runner who gives back to his native country. My husband's company matches charitable donations, so that year we gave about $800.

There have been times where I've picked up a $20 bill I found and thought, "I need a new pair of socks." No. It has to go in the running jar.

It probably sounds really dorky, but usually I run alone so I get really excited when I find money. It breaks up the monotony and pulls me out of whatever mental fog I might be in. It brings me back to the present. It doesn't matter if it's a penny, a quarter, or a $10 bill: I always get happy. Sure, it might be just a nickel, but it's ten cents with the company match.

—SAMANTHA (Wants to attempt a sprint triathlon. "Don't own a bike, and only own bikinis, so not sure when this will happen.")

IN HER SHOES: HANGING BY A FENCE

In the back of my neighborhood, there is a tall, swinging-gate-type of fence I frequently squeeze my body through to get to the tiny neighboring town of San Antonio. The top of the six-foot-high fence is strung with barbed wire so I usually squeeze through the gate, which just has a length of chain and a padlock keeping it shut. I've learned if I push one side of the locked, swinging gate, I can easily squat down and wiggle my body between the opening. I've done it tens, if not hundreds, of times.

On this day, though, there is something different about the fence. Later, I found out the owner had tightened the chain around the gate because he'd heard people were squeezing through.

But I don't know this fact as I lace my fingers through the gate and give it a hefty push. I squat and shove a leg through, wiggle and squirm so the first half of my bottom is through and the other half . . . is not. I'm stuck. One leg in San Antonio. The other out.

Nice one, Melissa, I think, *effing brilliant.* I wonder how hard my good pals at Pasco Fire Rescue are going laugh about this one. They are all too familiar with assisting my family from the many disasters my four sons have created. This predicament should really put them over the edge.

I start wiggling. I wiggle a little. I wiggle a lot. I wiggle some more. I bend; I twist; I grunt; I laugh; I tear up; I huff; I puff; I twerk. It feels like hours pass. And, then, in a move so badass it would have made Miley proud, my right butt cheek joins its counterpart.

Praise the Fence Gods: I am unstuck!

Then it hits me: I'm on the wrong side. I am back on the *inside* of my neighborhood. I should just run home, where there is air conditioning, Doritos, and reality TV waiting for me.

Then I look at the top of the fence. The part with the barbed wire. I totally think I can take it. I really need to run. Like, I.really.really.have.to.run. I have to run so my sons can live to see another sunrise, if you know what I mean.

I walk over to a grassy patch and dig my shoe into the fence. One shoe in, then the other, one leg over, then . . . one leg not over. I'm stuck again. Worse, my running shorts catch a sharp edge on the tip of the fence wire, leaving me to use all of my upper-body strength, which is roughly equal to that of a nine-year-old boy, to keep my lady parts away from the sharp top of the fence.

This cannot be happening to me. After four C-sections, I thought I had escaped ever having to undergo an episiotomy, but now it appears I am about to give myself one. Right here. On this damn fence.

Then the thought flashes through my mind: There is a likely chance this whole episode is on film. Recently the owner of the empty lakefront lot near this fence told me he had put up security cameras to keep an eye on his acreage. He was concerned about trespassers jumping the fence gate. Not only am I not going to get my miles in, my next stop is going to be jail.

Hold up: *three hots and a cot?* Maybe not so bad for a weary BAMR.

After a few minutes, I somehow heave myself over the fence—delicate bits still intact—and manage to get in my (much-needed) long run.

—MELISSA (While her then-baby napped, she put the baby monitor at the end of her driveway, then ran up and down the street, stopped to listen, and repeated the cycle for as long as possible. No fences involved.)

IN HER BRA: LOCKING AND LOADING THE LADIES

My chest has increased in size with each of my two kids. Twelve years ago, I used to be a pert 36C. Then I had my son and Mother Nature decided I was a great milk producer. I moved from a C cup to a D. Still, I could still find the over-the-head bras that fit. I'd get a little bit of bounce, but nothing too bad.

With my daughter, who is about to turn two, I entered a whole new "you can't buy something off the, ahem, rack" scenario. First, I tried on my pre-pregnancy bra, and it was like trying to stuff a sleeping bag into a sandwich bag. Wasn't gonna happen.

My 36D turned into a 36G. And not perky 36Gs. *National Geographic* 36Gs.

I'd heard a lot of people wear two sports bras for support, so I tried the double-boulder-holder thing. Post-run, it's hard enough being all sweaty to get one bra off, let alone two. Plus, even with two, my chest basically traveled at least twice as far as I did. With each step, my rack bounced up and down or side to side; the movement added to the overall tiredness I, who was already out of shape, felt.

So I went shopping. I would find a bra that fit the cups but it didn't give me support around the band. I found a style that fit around the band but created cleavage city: Everything was right at neck level. I'm sure there are people going out to a dance club who like everyone looking at their rack, but I'm not running in a nightclub.

I did test drive 100-yard dashes in the store and I thought I'd give myself a black eye. Very, *very* uncomfortable.

I finally found a solution with bras that have the fatter straps and extra padding on the shoulder. It's not really attractive—I used to call them Old Lady Padding—but those features help distribute the weight of my globes. I ordered the bras from Nordstroms. Even with free shipping and free returns, each bra costs 60 bucks, so I only own two. But those bras are worth every penny.

—LISA (Served her then-nursing daughter "margaritas" after a run: Her babe was too
hungry to wait for her mom to shower, so she was rimmed with salty sweat.)

IN HER SHOES: LEADING THE PACK

I'm competing in my second sprint triathlon in San Francisco, the now-defunct Golden Gate Triathlon. The half-mile swim is in the San Francisco Bay; the 10- or 15-mile bike is around city neighborhoods; and the 5K run traverses the hilly Presidio.

The swim went well despite choppy water and churning legs, and I make a good transition out of the Bay onto the bike. This is where the trouble starts.

I'm in the front third and with a small pack of cyclists who are all playing off one another. There are a crazy number of turns and unknown streets through small neighborhoods for a reasonable bike course. I'm with my friends for about the first 15 minutes, but we've all agreed to do our own race. After about 25 more minutes, the pack suddenly seems very small—and I'm in a pack of guys. I'm expecting people to be catching up with me at any moment, but the men all seem confident.

The bike portion seems long enough while we're riding, but as we are heading down the final downhill turns into the Presidio, I start to think something has gone wrong. I don't have a bike computer to let me know for sure. Near the transition area, I hear people cheering and yelling, "First woman! First woman!" Over a loudspeaker, I hear "Phebe Kiryk of Berkeley!"

Then I see my husband jumping up and down and running to meet me at the transition. I know I am in big trouble, because there is no way I am the first woman! He keeps yelling, "You got it! Go!" He and his friends seem so excited my inner athlete has finally come out. There is so much commotion and cheering for me to go-go-go, I just dump my bike, get on my running shoes, and charge out the gate.

But once I'm on the run course by myself, it feels like cheating. I'm pumped on adrenaline and running at a personal-best pace, yet I realize I cannot come in first. One woman passes me, and gives me a sideways look that says, I've never seen *you* before in the top finishers. But I do not want to give up. Even though I am sure I had gotten off-course on the bike, I have to finish.

Then I spy a green porta-potty on the course; I brilliantly decide to hop in to hide for a few minutes to allow more women to catch up. So there I am, in my swimsuit and running shoes, waiting for what seems like forever—but it is only like five or seven minutes.

I reemerge and finish the run, now surrounded by a few more competitors.

I come in fourth but immediately disqualify myself to keep the race right. Still it is my most exciting race ever: For those few minutes, I was a celebrity athlete!

—PHEBE (Admits this is one of those stories her family loves to tell again and again.)

IN HER SHOES: WINNING A MARATHON AT AGE FORTY-ONE

After swimming competitively from ages eight to twenty-two, I was completely burned out on stopwatches and times and tenths-of-a-second. So, at age twenty-two, I decided to train for a marathon because I wanted a race in which the goal was simply to finish. I ran the 1994 Chicago Marathon and loved it. I ran Boston the next spring, then Chicago again, and I kept running marathons for fitness and fun and the experience, never focusing very much on speed or times.

Fast forward to age thirty-nine, right after my fourth—and final—baby turned one. I finished breastfeeding and felt like my body was mine again for the first time in years. We had just moved to Portland, Oregon, and I found myself surrounded by fun, fast women who were racing, not just running. For the first time ever, I was inspired to set a time goal. Thanks to increased mileage, speedwork, and an aging body, I had a whole host of injuries, but I learned to be more careful with my hydration and nutrition, to foam roll, and to make time for bodywork appointments. Eventually, I ran faster than I ever had.

On the starting line of the 2013 Vancouver USA Marathon, I remember my goal: to break three hours. I am in third place for about the first half, and I pass the woman in second in mile 13. Pretty soon after that, around miles 14 or 15, when spectators start yelling out "second woman!" and "The first woman is dying! You look so much stronger!" I kind of have an idea there is a good chance I could catch the girl in the lead!

After a couple more miles, I start seeing her. Right around mile 20, there is a huge hill and I can see her walking up it, and I'm feeling good. I can catch her. I pass her around mile 21 or 22. I don't say anything to her until after the race, when we are interviewed together for a TV station.

I don't think the runners I've passed are going to come back and catch me, but when you're first in those last few miles, you feel like the rabbit being chased, whether that's the reality or not. I didn't go into the race thinking, *I really want to win this*, but now that I'm in that position, I don't want to get caught. I can't slow down. I've got to keep going. Everything hurts and I just want to stop and be done.

I am exhausted from maintaining a sub-7-minute pace for nearly three hours. For the last 22 miles, I had put it all out there to run the fastest splits I could. At the end, it takes everything I have to hold on to my pace. My stomach hurts. My legs want to stop, and I'm getting a headache. I want to be done.

I am on pace to hit 2:59. I turn the final corner and I can see the finish line. For the last 200 yards, the pain goes away. All of a sudden I can start sprinting again. But I wish that part would last a little longer because I'm finally enjoying the feeling of I'm going to finish. I'm reaching this goal. And I'm winning this race.

Breaking the tape is super cool. I'm totally wiped and elated—and feel huge relief that it's over. I have an involuntary smile. An announcer puts a microphone in my face. Friends and family are along the side of the chute. I go say hi. I pull my kids over the barriers and we get pictures taken. Then it just turns into a party.

—JEN (Clocked a blazing 2:58:54.)

IN HER SHOES: BRINGING UP THE REAR

I started running when I was thirty-nine years old and had just lost sixty pounds. For my second 5K, my running partner, Deb, and I participated in a small race during my alma mater's homecoming weekend.

Most of the final mile was along a parade route, and the race was scheduled to conclude about a half-hour before the parade began—a great idea unless you are slow and new to racing, which Deb and I both are. Most of the other runners are college kids, who quickly leave us in their dust. After a half-mile, there are only about five people around us.

I had pressed the wrong button on my GPS, so we have no idea what pace we are running. There is one girl about ten yards in front of us. We keep reeling her in and passing her, but that is her cue to pass us.

The final mile of the course is along the parade route—and it is lined with people. They are clapping. But it wasn't too enthusiastic clapping—they just want the parade to start. One kid along the way yells at us, "You're the *last* ones!" I am embarrassed and pretty discouraged—and worn out. I am ready to be done, but I can't see the finish line. Each block, I think it should be the final one.

There is no way I can go faster. My legs are tired of moving and my whole body is ready to stop. A friend who finished in 24 minutes comes out to cheer us on the final stretch. When we cross the finish line, there are people milling around but they've stopped yelling out times. Deb and I are the last people to cross the line.

When I see our finish time, however, I realize we've PR'd by about 5 minutes, and our discouragement turns to genuine excitement. Now I just make sure races I enter don't end on parade routes.

—KATE (until age 39, she "avoided running at all costs. In high school I was the track timer so I could be on the team and not run.")

IN HER SHOES: REMEMBERING MY FIRST TWENTY-SECOND INTERVAL

After 5 minutes of walking with my beginning running program with ladies from church, my first running interval came up: 20 seconds. I was just so excited to be doing it—and it wasn't as hard as I thought it would be. Tears came to my eyes. I was like, *I'm actually running!* Being very overweight, in my late forties, and a cancer survivor—I had non-Hodgkin's lymphoma at age thirty-nine—the odds were against me.

I also thought, *Oh, I'm not as tired as I thought I'd be.* Before I started this workout, I thought I'd be too wiped out to do more than one running interval but I wasn't. A minute's rest was all I needed.

The next running interval came up and I could do it! I did it again! And again! And again! It was like "Oh! This is so great!" It was just a shock. I was elated.

The next day I wanted to do the same workout again, but the leader of the group said, "Your body needs to rest." I wanted more, though.

Those 20 seconds changed my life. *Hey, I'm a runner!* I thought. *I never dreamed that would happen.*

—SUE (A man from her church gave her his 5K medal when the race she did ran out of them. "I cherish that medal.")

IN HER SHOES: MISSING A THIRTY-HOUR CUTOFF

I feel decent for the first 50 miles of the Leadville 100, an out-and-back trail race in the Colorado Rockies. Around mile 45, the first time I top 12,600 feet and go through Hope Pass, I hit the "Hopeless" aid station. It's not an official station, but every year a bunch of race supporters manage to create it by using llamas to carry all of the supplies near the top. Everybody *oohs* and *ahhs* over the ramen noodle soup. It tastes really good to me, and I feel like I can keep going.

The second time I have to get over Hope Pass, I slowly start to die. The backside of Hope is extremely steep. I struggle the entire way and constantly fight the urge to stop entirely and take a break. I don't take any breaks, but my pace is extremely slow. It probably takes 30 minutes to cover a mile.

My body is like, *Whoa. What are you asking me to do?* I have no energy left, and I start chasing race cutoffs; you have to be at a certain mile by a certain time, or the organizers pull you from the course.

On one flat section of the race around mile 75, my pacer, Julie, encourages me to run. I tell her I'll try, but to give me a minute to start going before she starts running. I take three cleansing breaths, which really seem to help, and pick it up. I feel like I'm really moving. Then Julie walks up beside me and says, "Um, Katie, I think you were actually just walking faster."

I get to the last aid station, 13.5 miles from the finish, with 6 minutes to spare before the cutoff. The aid station guy says, "Look, you can make the thirty-hour cutoff, but you're going to have to run around the lake." I think to myself: There's just no way I can run.

The trail around Turquoise Lake is a single-track trail. On Saturday, when the race started, I ran around the lake because at that point, the single-track was no big deal. But it's Sunday morning now, and, after already having 85 miles under my belt, I know I can't. Every step I take, especially on the downhill, sharp pain radiates from my ankles up my calves. I am too afraid to take any painkillers—and it's a good thing because my body is totally whacked out. I am puffy and retaining water. I haven't consumed enough salt and that, combined with being on my feet for nearly thirty hours, has really made my feet and legs swell. (When I'm weighed at the finish, I discover I have gained four pounds.)

I have a pretty bad blister on the bottom of one of my feet, but that pales in comparison to the pain in my ankles and the fatigue in my entire body. The blister is a nice distraction. If I can focus on that pain on the bottom of my foot, it takes my mind off the rest of my body for a bit.

Although my support crew tells me I only have to do 14-minute miles, that feels impossible to me right now. But I know I have to finish this race. Plus, there are people still behind me. I'm not the last one. So I just keep going. The final 5 miles are uphill, which doesn't bother me at this point.

My sister Annie is pacing me, and she keeps looking at me. Up and down. A full head-to-toe inspection. The nurse in her is trying to figure out what is happening to me. In my mind, there is nothing we can do anyway, so I prefer she wouldn't look at me that way—and tell her so. She is mostly compliant, but occasionally, I see her checking me out out of the corner of her eye. I yell at her, "Would you stop that?" She rattles on about my electrolytes or something and we keep walking. By this time, I've just accepted I'm probably not going to beat the cutoff.

Several times, I swear I see my husband, way off in the distance waving at me. I ask my sister, "Is that Tyler up there?" She says, "I don't think so." We get closer, and I realize there is nothing there. We go by a guy sitting down under a tree with a mile to go who lets the search and rescue truck pick him up. Never in a million years would I do that. Ever. I will crawl on my hands and knees.

When I see the finish line, organizers are rolling up the carpet but the clock is still out. I cross the finish at 30:28. Having my race "count" didn't really matter to me. I knew I wouldn't get a belt buckle, the prize for finishing in less than thirty hours. I am the last one to finish, but I am fine with that.

—KATIE (Got her belt buckle the following year.)

IN HER CAPRIS: STREAMING GALLANTLY

The first time I peed in my capris, I had my hand over my heart and, somewhere in the predawn darkness, a soprano was belting out "The Star-Spangled Banner." A steady rain was falling on my friends Julie and Ashley and me in starting corral B of the 2010 Portland Marathon.

In my last two marathons, I'd missed meeting my time goal by mere minutes—the amount of time I'd spent in a course-side porta-potty, pissing out some of the copious amounts of fluid I'd imbibed prerace. I vowed not to stop on this 26.2-mile go-round.

As cool raindrops splatter on my arms and the words, "Oh, say can you see," float through the air, I attempt a practice pee. It's been forty years since I last wore diapers, and every synapse and reflex in my body fights the instinct to relieve myself with fabric covering my lower half. My brain screams, "no," but my bladder—and sports ego—demands, "yes!"

I concentrate fiercely and bear down with my blanketed-in-fat lower abdominal muscles. "O'er the ramparts we watched were so gallantly streaming" fills the air as I'm able to squeeze out a few ounces of urine. My crotch immediately feels hot, and some lingering high-thigh chub-rub stings.

But practice makes perfect: Around Mile 15, when a true urge to purge hits, I am able to let loose on the fly. That time the warm ribbon of pee tickles my left inner thigh to my knee, petering out on my straining calf.

—SARAH (Otherwise known as SBS, who qualified for Boston, thanks, in part, to letting it fly.)

IN HER SHOES: FLYING THROUGH A 4:30 MILE

When I'm running as fast as I can, my brain is shut off so I can push my body into a place that isn't normal. What little thought I have is focused on finding that sweet spot of trying hard but not too hard. I have to stay loose and relaxed. Time kind of slows down; I can feel every step, every breath. Toward the end, it gets really hard and I just think, *legs go faster* so I can sprint at the end. The feeling of exhaustion doesn't come on until after I'm done.

—ROISIN (2008 Olympian in the Steeplechase)

IN HER SHOES: AVERAGING EIGHT-MINUTE MILES

Living in Cincinnati, I find myself in a Barnes & Noble in front of the running section. I see a book titled something like *Run a Marathon in 99 Days*. I always wanted to run a marathon—not sure why—and the timing is mostly right. I only have 90 days until the Flying Pig Marathon.

Not understanding what I am doing, I sign up for the race, jump right in, and skip the first week of training. Caveat: I had never, ever run. Ever. I start run-walking and work my way up.

The Friday night before the marathon, my mom calls and says I need to get back home to Rochester, New York. My brother is dying from a cancer we'd just found out he had, and he's in the hospital. There are no flights until Sunday afternoon. I make the decision to run the marathon. I believe I can finish and make it to the plane on time.

At mile 12, I sit down on the edge of the road and start sobbing. Uncontrollably melting down. For an hour. Finally, another female runner sees me and asks what's wrong. After she hears my story, she says, "You have to get on that plane. You can't run if you're crying, but you can't cry if you're running." She physically pulls me up and holds my hands until I start walking. As I calm down, I start running, and we pick up the pace.

I do some math—the only running math I've ever done correctly, by the way—and realize I'll have to pick the pace up even more to make it to the plane on time. Once I start running again, something in me snaps. I become angry at myself for sitting down and crying for an hour. Really? Who has the hydration, in the middle of a marathon, to cry for sixty minutes?

I know I have to run faster than I've ever run before. Incidentally, it never occurs to me to quit. Once I start running again, I'm not about to let all the training and questioning about my choice to run the marathon be for nothing. I never think about hailing a cab or taking the SAG wagon.

My first miles back aren't so hard. I have the drive, determination, and, after the hour off, relatively fresh legs and lungs. I systematically pick off every person walking in front of me and then every person run-walking. This gets me easily to mile 18. At this point, it's late enough in the race that organizers are starting to tear down the aid station. Adding to the downer vibe is the location: an industrial part of town with no one—and I mean *no one*—cheering me on. It's mentally tough and my hips are starting to complain about the speedy pace. I decide to ignore it and deal with the consequences later.

My mind keeps swinging back to my brother and if I made the right choice to run. Then it goes blank as I try to run even faster with more and more physical pain. The last mile or two goes over the bridge from Kentucky back into Cincinnati. I realize the SAG wagon is catching me and that I really have to push if I'm going to make my plane.

I give it everything I have on that bridge and on the road to the start of the finish chute. I feel empty, spent, and drained. I feel like my body is just a shell where there is nothing left. It is everything I can do to put one foot in front of the other.

I cross the finish line and, incredibly, as I'd skipped aid stations to save time and am not very well hydrated, burst into tears. Again.

Even though I had planned on doing 11-minute miles for the entire race, I later find out I'd run 8-minute miles for the back half of the marathon.

My husband picks me up at the finish line. I get in the car immediately—no cool down, no shower, no change of clothes—and get on the plane.

I make it back in time to say good-bye to my brother.

—JENNIFER (Tossed her running shoes after that marathon and didn't run again for a decade, until after her second child was born.)

IN HER SHOES: RUNNING FEARLESS

In 1975, I arrived at the Boston Marathon starting line utterly fearless. I had done so much home-work, including 27-mile runs every Sunday, I was beyond ready to go. Once I was running, it was like the road came to meet me. I had my goal paces written on my arm, but I couldn't figure how to match them to my watch, so I just went.

Climbing hills, I felt like I was a champagne cork coming out of a bottle. I was running without pain or effort, I would look up and think, "How did I get to this neighborhood so quickly?" For the whole 26.2 miles, I had a breeze in my face. I was running fast enough to create my own breeze.

—KATHRINE (Clocked a 2:51 eight years after her 1967 history-making Boston Marathon appearance, which was 4:20. "Hard work really works.")

IN HER SHOES: RACKING UP FOURTEEN-MINUTE MILES

I ran my first half-marathon a year ago, and I'm currently training for my third half. I consistently run a 14-minute mile in my longer races. It takes me a little over three hours to run a half-marathon. I can't go fast, but I can go far—and I always finish.

I'll never be a competitive racer, but I really enjoy the atmosphere of being on the course on race day. I like feeling the adrenaline and the camaraderie of people who have put in the same number of miles in training. It feels good knowing we've all put in a lot of sweat to get to the same place. All the races I've done have good spectators and I feed off that energy. I've been lapped by full marathoners on some courses, but I never feel judged by anyone on the race course. I've never felt "less than" as a slower runner. And I've never felt anything but support from faster runners.

I normally run at a conversational pace, but on race day, there's a harder pace. I can breath, and I can talk in two or three word clips. But there's definitely more push, more *oomph* on race day.

I have a few favorite songs, like "Whoomp! (There It Is)," that song from the 1990s. When I feel myself dragging, I'll put a song on repeat. Or if I'm running with a certain friend of mine, I tell her she needs to share a story from her days in the Peace Corps to take my mind off my fatigue.

I am a runner, but I line up toward the back of the race pack. I'm usually with a lot of power walkers—those are the people I like to pass in the final few miles. It boosts my morale when I pass people. I think, "I'm going for it!"

—KERRY (Named the pair of shoes she wore in her first half-marathon Lois and Flo because "I felt if they had names, they would carry me faster!")

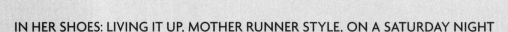

IN HER SHOES: LIVING IT UP, MOTHER RUNNER STYLE, ON A SATURDAY NIGHT

I'm not able to get out for my long training run for my first, post-baby half-marathon in the morning because I have two small kids—at the time they were two years old and six months old—and my husband is at work all day. I need to run 10 miles.

So I do what any mother runner in my situation would do: jump on the treadmill in July in our un-air-conditioned basement at 9 p.m. after both kids are in bed. It's like a dungeon down there. There's nothing to look at but the '70s-era paneled walls. All I have is music and prayers it will be done soon. I cover the treadmill readout with a towel. If I have the blinking light that goes around the virtual track staring at me, the time d.r.a.g.s.

Surprisingly, the first couple of miles aren't too bad. Partly it's because I don't think I fully believe I am actually going to run 10 miles on the treadmill. Usually I do about half of a required run and call it a day. So some misguided optimism helps me there.

After those first miles, I keep thinking, "This is just one run. You can just stop and do it another day." But I figure I am there. I already have the rank-stank odor going. I might as well just finish it. I promise myself for the next mile I'm not going to think about the fact I'm running that mile.

So I keep saying to myself, "This is what my life has become. The 20-year old me would be at the bar, dancing, having fun on a Saturday night, and I'm wallowing in my own sweat on a treadmill with my kids sleeping upstairs."

When I'm done, I feel disgusting because I've been running through pudding for the last hour and a half. I didn't think it was humanly possible to be that saturated after a run. I seriously contemplate throwing my running shirt out; it's not worth salvaging.

At my husband's request, I take a cold shower before getting into bed. This is one of the few runs where I am able to shower right after because usually when I return from a morning run, my kids are ready to get the day's fun started.

So at least I have a clean body—and 10 miles in the books—going for me.

—STEPHANIE (Regularly reminds herself her chip times "aren't a reflection of my worth as a runner, mom, wife, or woman. I'm still a runner. A BAMR, to be precise.")

IN HIS SHOES: ROCKING THIS BABY

My six-year old son has cerebral palsy and is the most dedicated athlete I know.

I'd just run a benefit 5K for the special soccer team he plays on. Then there was a 1K for the kids. His older sister was so excited to do it, so of course, he's excited, too. He doesn't see he can't win anything yet. His state of mind is still: Hey, this is all mine. You can't take this from me.

That's awesome, by the way. We should all still feel like that.

My son crouches down at the start. I figure he's having problems standing and I'm trying to figure out what is wrong. But he's actually just getting into his runner's stance. He turns to me and says, "Mom. I'm gonna ROCK this baby."

"Yes, honey," I say. "Yes, you are."

And then I burst into tears after they start.

He rocked it. He rocked right over the finish line. He came in last, but the cheers for him were louder than for the people who came in first.

Now, before every run, I tell myself I'm gonna rock this baby.

—KRISTI (Advice for postpartum running: "Lots of compression gear, ladies.")

06

AMBITION:
Dream Big, Step Up

"I had been running for about a year, and I was training for my first half-marathon. I had to do a hot, hilly eight-miler by myself. Nobody was home when I slogged up the hill to my house. When I stopped at my driveway, I cried tears of joy and relief. I couldn't believe I had just done that all by myself."

—ELLEN

WHO NEEDS PRADA? I'VE GOT COACH.
by Bethany Meyer

I love running for the way it leans out my body, which is curvy from head to toe. I love it for the way it nurtures my friendships, which sometimes suffer when the balance tips to favor my family of five males (one husband, four sons). I love it for its methodical ease of putting one foot in front of the other to get from here to there. I love it for its complicated side, that intangible force that pulls me to wake before sunrise to log miles or to tap into a part of me I never knew existed to complete a grueling workout or cross a finish line. And I love it for the way it quiets my mind, which is typically so jumbled with all things Mom.

Where are my library books? Is my basketball uniform clean? Is Dad coming to my game? Where's my retainer? Am I going to Jack's birthday party? Did you get a gift? Can I have a playdate? He's had two playdates; when is it my turn for a playdate? Can I buy this app? What should I wear? Does my suit need dry cleaning? Where's my belt? Are we out of chicken nuggets? Can I buy hot lunch tomorrow? Can you make cheeseburgers tonight? Did I turn on the crockpot? Did I turn off the iron? Did you take your medicine? Has anyone fed the cat?

It's the thinking I do—the thinking for all of us—that does me in.

So I run.

When I began running ten years ago, I looked to Hal Higdon for my training plans. Bless his heart, Hal never let me down. Then I had success with the plans in *Train Like a Mother*. Sarah and Dimity's "Own It" plans are a certified ass-kicking. Then my friend Schuyler asked me to run a Ragnar Relay with her. I agreed. Before I knew what it was.

What is this Ragnar Relay business? I wondered. So I Googled it. It is a 200-mile race. A team event. Each team has twelve runners. Each runner hits the course three times to help the team complete 200 miles. There is a runner on the course at all times, which equates to little sleep and running at odd hours for everybody. You run 6 miles, jump into a cramped van in your swampy running clothes, drink chocolate milk for recovery, wait eight or ten hours, then do it again. And again.

Now, I'm no elite runner. I don't expect to place in my age group, even in small races. But I also didn't want to flail on the Ragnar course. The notion of racing three different times in one race had both me and Schuy stumped.

No one—not Hal, not the Mother Runners, not anybody else we Googled—had a training plan for a race as unorthodox as Ragnar.

We needed someone to create a training plan. Actually, we needed someone to think for us. We needed a running coach.

As luck would have it, my husband was in the throes of a bromance with his best running friend, who had recently trained him to run a 5K in under twenty minutes. It had been my husband's long-time goal to break 20:00. He'd come close in the past, but didn't achieve his goal until he put his training into someone else's hands. And he chose very capable hands. His friend—and coach—had won the Philadelphia Public League Cross-Country Championship in high school. Philadelphia cross-country runners compete at Belmont Plateau. Will Smith put Belmont Plateau on the musical map in his song "Summertime." But in the running community, they're singing a different tune: Belmont Plateau is one of the most respected—and one of the toughest—cross-country courses in the Northeast.

Naturally, Schuy and I Googled our potential coach's high school times. That made us *really* nervous about enlisting his help. The man was way out of our league, running-wise.

Would he critique our strides? Because the idea of that made me uneasy. Two words: butt jiggling. Would he expect us to run six days a week? Because that is too many for me. Would we have to sacrifice our beloved strength training and yoga while we trained with him? You may not mess with my OM. Would he even want to work with us? Because breaking 20:00 in a 5K is not in either of our wheelhouses. Never has been, never will be.

Still, we met with the man who'd mentored my husband.

Nervously.

He asked for a commitment of four days a week of running. With a focus on Ragnar, he talked about training our bodies to run on fatigued legs, which meant running doubles as race day approached. He encouraged us to continue our strength training and yoga. After one conversation, we were sold. My husband's BRF became our Coach.

When training began, Coach eased us into it. Schuy was in decidedly better shape than I was. She'd run two half-marathons recently. I hadn't run a race in a year and was just coming off crutches for a sprained ankle, which was still swollen and had little range of motion. "Easy" was the only gear I had fifteen weeks before race day.

The training plans Coach created for us were similar for the first month. We communicated via spreadsheet on a smartphone app, which was perfect for our busy lifestyles. He asked we do the work, then provide feedback after every run.

How far did you go?

How long did it take you?

What was the temperature?

What time of day did you run?

What shoes did you wear?

How did you feel?

Comments about the run?

My comments section read like a diary.

Today I ran six miles at 2PM. It was 92 degrees. I HATE running in the heat. Absolutely loathe it. I usually stop running altogether in the summer. That's how much I hate running in the heat. I was working much harder than the time on my watch said. Maybe my watch is broken. I'm serious. I never hit a groove. My legs didn't feel it. My music sucked. It was a terrible run from start to finish. Blah. Blah. BLAH.

The next entry read . . .

Soooo, I got my period today. Which is probably why I felt altogether like shit during yesterday's run. You don't have any sisters, do you? Sorry. Oversharing. Never mind. In related news, sometimes it sucks to be a girl. Today I logged 4 miles and I felt uh-may-zing. Crushed it. Too legit to quit. And, yes, I'm dancing like MC Hammer in my kitchen as I type this.

I've logged my food in the past. *I ate a spinach salad with 1 tablespoon of Italian dressing. I skipped the bacon. I rewarded myself for skipping the bacon with one chocolate chip cookie. Because it was homemade and still warm. I felt guilty about that, but not so guilty that I won't do the same thing again tomorrow.* Keeping a food journal was more exhausting than skipping the bacon, and I usually quit after five or so meals.

But there was something therapeutic about logging those training miles after every run. It was evidence, in my own words, that I was growing more powerful and race-ready every week.

The training miles also forced me to be present during my runs in a way I've never before been. Running with friends has always meant shifting my body to autopilot and catching up on one another's lives. Running alone has meant finding just the right music or podcast to mirror the intensity of my workout. My spreadsheet was my reminder to tune in, not out. In order to get the full benefit of all Coach had to teach me, I owed it to both of us to pay attention. In the heat. On the hill. Once a day. Twice a day. *How does this feel? Right now? In this spot? Coach wants to know. I need to be able to tell him.*

Managing everyone's demands simultaneously isn't the hardest part of being a mom. That juggling act eventually becomes second nature. If I am juggling ten balls in the air, more often than not, I'm not giving them my full attention. I'm looking for that eleventh ball just around the corner. Also, I'm wondering if chicken breasts are on sale this week. Because I'm Mom, I'm always looking forward. I am the anticipator of needs. That makes being present my greatest challenge. I was invested when Coach trained me. Engaged. Present. I showed up, body and mind. I stopped anticipating what was around the corner, and I was able just to be.

As the days rolled into weeks, our training became more specific and individual. Schuy learned her first leg of Ragnar would be a trail run. *Lucky duck.* Mine would begin at the bottom of a steep, 2-mile incline. *Mother humper.*

Ten weeks from race day, there was a definite shift in the intensity of our running. Our plans morphed from easy runs into *Coach-cannot-be-serious-about-this* runs.

I texted Schuy one evening, "Did you get your plan for this week?"

She replied, "I'm on the track. Intervals. I've never run this fast. I'm nervous. I don't think I can do it. You?"

"Four to eight quarter-mile hill repeats. Then a 1-mile tempo run. Uphill. Followed by four to eight quarter-mile hill repeats. I vomited in my mouth reading it. Coach is insane."

I read the details of that workout over and over. I wrote it on my hand in ink so I didn't forget it in the midst of running it. I chose my music carefully. Packed more water than usual. Drove, with butterflies in my stomach, the two miles from my house to the run. I'd been an athlete all my life. I'd been running for a decade. I'd trained seriously for races in the past. I'd given birth four times, for Pete's sake! But I didn't know if I had it in me to do this workout. I was psyching myself out completely.

I sat in my minivan, grasped the steering wheel tightly, inhaled the scent of stale Goldfish crackers, and put on my game face. "Coach believes I can do it," I said aloud.

And so I did it. Damn, it hurt. But I did it.

It was Coach's unspoken faith in me that got me through the toughest hill workout I've ever done. I mean, he wouldn't have given it to me if he didn't think I could do it, would he? Would he?

I could hardly wait to text Schuy: "I did it! Hardest hill workout ever, done!"

Her reply was immediate. "OMG! I'm so excited for you! Guess what? I did my intervals. And I was able to run them faster than Coach told me to run! I can't believe it! I'm so excited!"

I typed: "Congratulations!! Coach is going to yell at you for going too fast. But semantics. Yay!!"

I typed my feedback to Coach wearing a dopey grin on my face. And when he replied, "Nice work, Meyer. That was a killer workout. You nailed it. Proud of you," that dopey grin became a permagrin.

Then I spied my next hill workout scheduled for two short weeks later.

There is a beast of a hill, just shy of a mile, right by the entrance to my kids' school. It's the kind of hill that makes you die a little bit inside when you raise your eyes and see it is steepest at the top. I ran that hill with a friend while she trained for the Boston Marathon. She always ran it faster than I did, and I'd often stop and walk part of it. I'd shout, "Boston! Woohoo!" at her retreating back as she climbed, and I'd fiddle with my music, looking for the "Rocky" theme to inspire me to pick up my pace. (*Yo, Adrian, I'm from Philly, what can I say?*)

Naturally, Coach put me on that hill for repeats. It was an unseasonably warm ninety degrees the early afternoon of my run. Coach had instructed me to warm up with a slow mile, and then hit that dreaded hill. Four times. In. A. Row. During the workout, I wanted to stop and walk like I had in the past. But I wouldn't let myself walk. Because this time I was accountable and present. My running spreadsheet was my confessional, and if I walked, I'd be forced to admit my sins. "Bless me, Father, for I have sinned. Gee, that hill is steep. Maybe after four Hail Marys and three Our Fathers, I'll get it next time." Not a chance. I wouldn't write it. As I'd been doing for weeks, I put my head down and did the work. And, Coach's plan was working. Because I ran it in negative splits.

Being accountable to Coach meant demanding more of myself. Although it sounds harsh, the demands didn't leave me feeling drained. They actually gave me confidence. As Mom, I'm a lifter of spirits, encouraging my family as they navigate work, school, and relationships. While they support me in return, training with Coach was like having my own little cheerleader, one who is not rooting for me, then asking for a ham sandwich. And there is something to be said for encouragement that comes sans a request for deli meat. It feels more authentic.

After fifteen weeks of training, we arrived at Ragnar with our legs and lungs pumped and our prerace jitters low. Coach had asked us to trust him, and we had. Ragnar wound up being the most amazing race experience I've ever had. For thirty-six hours, I forgot I lived in the real world.

I existed in an alternate universe where my van-mates became my family, and our biggest stress was whether we could hit a Chipotle before running again. I loved every minute. Even those spent climbing the dreaded hill.

The week after the race, I was tired but euphoric. I kept in close touch with my new Ragnar family, reminiscing about our favorite memories over social media. Eager to maintain my level of fitness, I laced up my sneakers for a run, checked my spreadsheet to see what Coach had assigned, and found a giant goose egg.

Absolutely nothing.

Panic! *How far should I go? How fast? Tempo? Long and slow? Hills? Intervals?*

It was as though I'd forgotten how to run without Coach thinking for me. That nimble little minx had become invaluable. He had become my personal Dear Abby for all things running. So Schuyler and I kept him around.

His presence in my life is the best gift he could have given me. Better than a new GPS. Better even than a PR. Coach gives me confidence, accountability, and the elusive ability to be present.

And he gives me relief. The relief I didn't know I needed. The relief that, as long as his spreadsheets are around, I will have one less thing to think about.

TAKE IT *From* A MOTHER
WHAT IS YOUR PROUDEST RUNNING MOMENT?

"I wanted to run 10 miles before my one-year 'runiversary,' and I did it two weeks ahead of schedule. My legs felt strong, and I floated on the pride of my first double-digit run for many, many days afterward."

— KATE (Started running when she felt like "her entire life revolved around filling sippy cups, shuffling laundry, and negotiating with terrorists. I mean, toddlers.")

"Finishing Cleveland's Finest 5K neck and neck with a Marine, all while my kids and husband watched! My 'Chariots of Fire' moment. She held me off for the first two-and-one-half miles, and we crossed next to each other. After the finish, she admitted the sound of me behind her kept her running so fast."

—JENNIFER (Has regretted, more than once, not looking at a race course map or weather forecast.)

"Truthfully, I was disappointed in my marathon time, but I just can't help but be proud I did it. To believe I could was a huge mental hurdle for me—and to prove it to myself was a giant accomplishment."

—SARA (Holds "racing funds" garage sales.)

"Beating my husband—and getting a PR—in a 10K. I also got to fulfill my dream of having my girls watch me race; making a quick stop for hugs and kisses was priceless."

—ROBIN (Favorite time of day to run: "when somebody is watching the kids.")

"The first time I placed in a 5K, which was my first race after my husband was deployed. I was shocked when they announced my name as third—and I've been gunning for a first ever since."

—RACHEL (Has racked up two firsts since then: one when there were only two people in her age group, and one in the "running with a dog" category. "Still striving for a legit first!")

"I gently pushed my sister, twelve years older than me, into running a half-marathon. I sent her a run/walk training plan and said, 'Do it!' She did! During the race, I refused to leave her, even though she encouraged me to. About mile five-and-a-half, she said, 'You probably saved my life. I was headed down a sedentary path I never would have left. Thank you.' I wanted to cry. She's still running today."

—KRISTY (Loves running in frigid weather. "The kind where you hack up ice after a run.")

"Twelve miles. In. A. Row."

—PAULA ("That's Not My Name" by the Ting Tings is the song that pumps her up.)

"I now have four marathons under my belt, but my proudest moment is still the first time I ran 2 miles without stopping."

—ALISON (While her husband doesn't "get" her running, her father-in-law is a runner so "he's accustomed to the eccentricities.")

"Winning a marathon—not my PR—as both first woman and first Master's woman at age forty-seven."

—ANGIE (BTW, her marathon PR, 3:07, was clocked at age forty-two. Her win was a 3:13.)

"Before I started running, I was diagnosed with and received treatment for a brain tumor. I ran a half-marathon—my first and only, so far—on the seventh anniversary of my brain surgery. I was completely overwhelmed with gratitude when I came around the last corner and saw my kids waiting there for me."

—EMILY (Proud moment number two: ran with her dad, who recently lost 100 pounds, for the first time last summer.)

"After shedding fifteen pounds in the past five months, I ran three PRs: 90 seconds off my 5K, 2 minutes off of my 10K, and 9 minutes off my half. Badass mother runner!"

—ANN (Hardest race moment: when her running buddy left her at mile 4 of a half-marathon. "We hadn't discussed the possibility of her taking off. We had talked about being there for each other.")

A SPECK THROUGH SPACE
by Katie Arnold

I am floating through Valles Caldera National Preserve. Less than one week from now, a wildfire will skirt the edges of this high, open bowl of grass and elk, an enormous, scooped-out shell of a 1.5-million-year-old volcano. But I'm the only thing burning here today. I'm just a body running, arms and legs firing in unison. My brain, along for the ride, devours everything in sight: chunks of glossy black obsidian strewn across the rocky double track, elk ribs bleached white, and far off in the grass, a lumpy skull. A dust devil swirls across the road ahead of me, a dirt-brown cyclone throwing its arms in the air. I have never seen anything as electric, or wondrous.

It's May 25, sometime before noon. I'm 20 miles deep into my first fifty-mile race, the Jemez Mountain 50-Mile Trail Run, in the high country west of Los Alamos, New Mexico. Rumored to be one of the toughest fifty-milers in the country, the race follows a long, mostly single-track loop that winds through foothills on the outskirts of Los Alamos before presenting the first of two climbs up 10,440-foot-high Pajarito Ski Resort in the mountains, then descending to the base lodge. From there, the course traverses high meadows and plunges down a loose, precipitous trail into the Valles Caldera.

Valles Caldera is actually seven *valles*, or grassy bowls, strung together like pearls. This section of the run is 12 miles of little-traveled, double-track Jeep roads, punctuated by two aid stations. The Caldera is a national preserve, and visitation is highly regulated. You can't just show up here on a normal Saturday and go running. Today, as every other day, you won't meet other visitors in this otherworldly place. In fact, the only humans I see, besides a few hardy volunteers, are a handful of other runners waging their own private negotiations with pain, fear, and pride.

I've been running for three hours and know what awaits me at the far end of the Caldera: a steep, hands-on-knees scramble up Pajarito for a second time. I've got 25 miles to go, and I'm too far in to turn back. I have to get out of the Caldera—and cover the same distance I've already gone—on my own.

It's taken me months to get here. All spring, I ran hills and mountains, experimented with nutrition and cross-training, put in long hours on the rolling flats to increase my speed. I mapped all-day, 35-mile solo runs in the backcountry near my home, dropped off my two daughters at school and ran all day, straight until pickup, when I'd show up sweaty with dirt-scuffed ankles, exhausted and ecstatic.

I've been a runner and outdoor athlete my whole life, but I only started racing ultras recently. Outdoor sports have always been an emotional, creative, and physical outlet for me, and nothing clears my mind and boosts my spirit like a few hours of hard exercise in the backcountry. I spent my twenties and early thirties riding mountain bikes, but after my first daughter was born, I turned more often to trail running. I could get in a great workout in less time than cycling, and didn't have to fuss over any gear; a baby was enough maintenance for me.

Then, two years later, in the course of three months, my second daughter was born and my father was diagnosed with cancer and died. When I finally emerged again from the fog of infancy and grief, I was desperate to reclaim my wild territory. My cravings for nature and wilderness were visceral and insatiable: For my sanity and creativity, I needed to go far and deep, but as a mother of an eighteen-month-old and a three-year-old, I had even less time to spare than before. The fastest way to go farther and wilder was to run.

Since running my first 50K, everything I've learned about ultrarunning I've gleaned through trial and error. I've never worn a heart-rate monitor. I don't have a coach or a training plan, and I don't track my stats or compete on Strava or even wear a watch. Maybe I'd be a faster runner if I did, but I prefer to train from the inside: by feel, by listening to my body, by running from the heart rather than from my head, by focusing on the private joy of moving through nature on my own two feet. When I do this, I invariably run faster, stronger, farther, and happier. I won my first two 50Ks with an ease that surprised me.

Despite this early, unexpected success, I started my second year as an ultrarunner freighted with worry. I've always had an active imagination, which comes in handy as a writer, but after becoming a mother and losing my father in that single season, my anxiety went into overdrive. Every possible thing in the world to worry about, I worried about. Caught in a cycle of postpartum, grief-induced anxiety, I envisioned terrible, improbable scenarios involving me and the people I loved most. Running in nature became a path through persistent grief, the surest cure for my anxiety, proof I was alive and strong. If I could knock off a 35-mile training day, reasoned my irrational mind, then I couldn't be dying of cancer.

On my best days on the trails, I stopped thinking and let my body take over. Legs flying, feet grounding me in the dirt, nose inhaling the sweet vanilla scent of summer ponderosas and hot pine needles baking in the sun, my racing brain was silenced for a few hours. The longer I ran, the more time I spent in that rare, peaceful place free of thoughts, doubts, fear. And the more I ran, the greater incentive I had to keep running.

But as I began training for my fifty-miler, I noticed anxiety beginning to creep in again. I came up with plenty of things to worry about. I was afraid of the distance—nearly double a 50K, my longest effort to date; of being stalked by mountain lions on my long, backcountry solo runs; of injuring myself and not being able to run. These, of course, were decoy fears invented by my brain to mask the real angst: What if my previous victories had been a fluke? What if I couldn't live up to my own mounting expectations? I'd been afraid of dying, but now I was afraid of losing. In some ways, they felt like the same thing to me.

I ran hundreds of miles in the mountains that spring, and I never crossed paths with anything larger than a squirrel. But I did get hurt. In late April, I overrode my body's signals, pushed through big, back-to-back runs, and strained my calf. It rose fat and swollen and angry, chastising me for trying to go too far, too steep, too fast. My mind snapped into action, busily trying to figure out everything. *How can I heal my leg without losing fitness? Should I run the race? What if I can't finish? Should I even start? Are humans meant to run this far?* I became a self-help junkie, desperate for any solution that might get me to the starting line, then the finish: foam rolling, taping, acupuncture, dry needling, Rolfing, omega-3 oil, massage, mountain biking, Arnica by the gallon, meditation. Some days I crammed a lightweight yoga mat into my pack, ran up the foothills outside of town, found a flat spot, and invented my own little backcountry yoga practice. The bumps of small pebbles and roots pressing through thin rubber into my back gave me an odd pleasure, reminding me of the real reason I run: to be outside, free, in nature.

Finally, a week before the race, sick of wondering whether I'd be able to do it, I decide the only way to find out was to try.

In the days leading up to the start, I make a deal with myself: If I want a shot at finishing the race with my injured calf, I have to pace myself. No racing, just running. So for the first 10 miles, I hold myself back, riding the heels of other runners and talking off my nerves. At 5 a.m., the full moon is sinking fast toward the lip of the Jemez Mountains looming just ahead, and the darkness keeps me from going too fast. Under the dim light of my headlamp, I spend the first 4 miles talking to the back of Jacob, a friend of a friend who, a week before the race, had sent me alarming messages on Facebook. "You need to keep it together in the Caldera," he warned, "because the climb out is brutal. It's like a sick joke."

Making Jacob talk to me is karmic payback for psyching me out, and our chatter reassures me I'm not running too fast. If I can carry on a conversation about where our four-year-olds take swimming lessons, maybe I'll improve my odds of getting out of the Caldera on both feet

After a while, Jacob stops talking and begins to pull away. He's a nuclear physicist. Maybe he knows something I don't about the science of endurance races: *Is it better to slow yourself down by talking or save your strength by shutting up?* My brain is so busy cartwheeling through scenarios and strategies and navigating the rock-strewn trail beneath my feet that I almost don't notice the brightening sky. But then I emerge from the trees into an open hillside burned several years ago in a forest fire, and I see it's daylight now. I shed my headlamp, and soon I crest a series of switchbacks just in time to watch the blazing disk of the sun clear the Sangre de Cristo Mountains behind me. Daybreak is a shot of optimism straight into the veins. I whoop to no one in particular, and dare to let myself think about my calf. It doesn't hurt.

Pretty soon I catch up to a guy from Oak Ridge, Tennessee, who tells me he was one of only two competitors to finish a brutal one-hundred-miler in Michigan last year; guys flaunting Western States buckles dropped like flies in the knee-deep soggy bog. We are running through the hot, charred remains of a forest fire; our footsteps spray a fine silty dust. He might as well be talking about another planet. "Have we started the big climb yet?" Oak Ridge asks me hopefully, but we are still in the cruisy rollers; the wretched slog up Pajarito Mountain rises ominously in the distance. It seems cruel to remind him we have to climb it twice, so I go for optimism over honesty. "Almost," I say, with a brightness I didn't think I'd feel.

The climb is one long switchbacking blur up the ski mountain. We pass in and out of thick stands of aspens and traverse steep, shaggy meadows, ski runs minus the snow. I catch a guy from Kansas who has stopped to take pictures, gazing appreciatively at the view of Los Alamos and the desert far below. I debate doing the same, but am too lazy to fish the phone from my race vest and worry that if I stop, I will never start again.

As relieved as I am when I crest Pajarito's summit, my brain is still calling the shots.

The conversation goes like this: "Slow down," brain says to body. "Trip now, and you could wreck yourself. You still have to run down this same mountain one more time. Save your speed for next time."

"But I want to go fast," body replies. "The faster I run, the sooner I'll see my husband, Steve, waiting at the bottom."

"You see that guy up ahead trip over that rock and fly through the air? See him hit the ground and bounce like a doll?" brain warns. "That could be you."

Body relents.

I manage to stay upright for the long, twisting descent, and pretty soon I'm at the ski lodge, roughly mile 18, where Steve and volunteers are ringing cowbells and hollering encouragement from the deck. I surrender my hydration pack for a refill, and place an order with Steve: two Advil, a handful of salt tabs for my pill pocket, headphones for my iPod, please. Due to my conservative pace, I'm half an hour behind where I estimated I'd be at this point, but I got here in one piece, and so far my legs are feeling strong. Self-restraint appears to be working.

"See you in twenty miles," I call over my shoulder to Steve, as I turn my music back on and pound across the wooden deck and into the forest again. For the first time all day—all season—I think I might actually pull it off.

I don't know if it's Gary Clark Jr. reminding me this is the life, the life, the life, the trail cutting through ponderosas alongside a grassy meadow, or seeing Steve, but on the 3-mile run out to Pipeline Aid Station, before we drop into the Caldera, something shifts. My brain detaches, a kite cut loose from its string. "You take it from here," it says to body. Suddenly I'm all legs, no thoughts. It's much easier this way—and faster.

At Pipeline, volunteers give me the once-over. "It's hot and exposed in the Caldera," they warn me. "No shade. Watch the descent into it. It's straight down and super loose." I have a hat and a hydration pack full of electrolytes and a couple of sticky orange slices in my hand. Good to go. They weren't exaggerating. It's sliding-on-your-butt steep. A half-mile at a thirty-five-degree angle. Clinging-to-trees steep. My socks and shoes fill with pebbles, dust, sand, dirt. I can feel the grit sloshing around inside, but my brain couldn't care less. Stopping isn't an option. My body just wants to run.

And then I'm in it—the Caldera—feet pinwheeling, body barely skimming the ground, senses inhaling every detail. The skeleton bones and dust devils. Runners I catch, then leave behind. Far in the distance, a shimmery pond I'd like to jump into, and miniature toy trucks propped up on a stage set, an aid station. The simplicity of my mission focuses me: Keep running. Get out of here. Twenty-three miles to the finish.

I'm a dot against grass and sky. Just like the runner far ahead of me, a black spot looping along the contours of the rough road. The runner, one of some 300 in the field, is slowly getting bigger. I'm gaining on him, if only by inches, just like I'm outpacing the two runners behind me, one step at a time. I feel outrageously lonely. I want to catch the runner just so I can shout out to him, "I'm so lonely!" but as he grows closer, I realize I don't actually want to talk to him, or anyone. Solitude is my fuel. We're in this together, but only I can get myself out of the Caldera.

At the halfway point, mile 25, a man at the aid station refills my hydration bladder and informs me it's 6.8 miles to the next one. I stuff my fists with orange slices, put my head down, and keep running. My pace is faster now than it's been the whole race. I've settled in. I'm cocooned in the Caldera, music fills my ears—Taylor Swift, Rufus Wainright, LMFAO. I'm party rocking in the house tonight. I'm no longer afraid. I've stopped thinking. I'm just running. I'm free.

Before I know it, 7 miles have disappeared beneath my feet. The backside of Pajarito Mountain looms up at me, the double track disappearing into grass and ponderosas, unmarked trail, unrelenting mountainside. Steve will be waiting on the other side to run the final 14 miles with me. All I have to do is climb out. Although my brain is on autopilot, I realize I already miss the scale and solitude, the simplicity of the task at hand. I almost don't want to leave.

Many people think running and racing is about speed, but really, it's about slowing down. You may be moving faster than you ever have on two legs, but in the quiet of prolonged effort, time stretches out, elongates. You listen to a song you've heard a hundred times before, and it sounds different. You hear it with your body, not your brain. You absorb everything around you: the waving grass, the elk high above you, trampling soot-black deadfall, the sweet orange slices that taste better than anything you've ever eaten in your life. Your mind drifts away; you're moving on instinct. You are transported without leaving your body. You are purely animal, unstoppable, fire storming across the forest, wild and alive.

Almost immediately after leaving the final aid station in the Caldera, I lose the course. The orange markers that have been leading us vanish. I slow to a walk and spend twenty minutes or more picking my way through tall grass, looking for the bright orange stick flags that have fallen over in the stiff spring wind or been trampled by elk. A small herd lumbers across the hillside in front of me, and I let them pass, more awed at their beauty than annoyed at being lost. I wait for two runners far below to catch up with me, and together we canvass the slope, looking for a sign we're on the right track. Eventually we see a single orange ribbon dangling from a branch, and we separate again, retreating into our private, silent worlds, bent into the mountain, making it out of the Caldera on our own.

At mile 36, after a long, wobbly-kneed descent down the ski area, I fling myself into the base-area aid station for the second time that day, so moved to see Steve and our daughters and the plate of red licorice that I nearly weep with happiness. For the final 14 miles, Steve paces me. With him, it's a different race: collaborative, no longer silent and solitary. As we lope through the white-hot lunar landscape of the recent forest fire, descending out of the Jemez and back toward town, he force-feeds me peanut-butter sandwich squares, points out wildflowers, and razzes me to run faster. I barely say a word back. I've moved so far past thinking: I'm just listening, absorbing, all senses firing. I drink in the hot blue sky, summer settling down on northern New Mexico, and feel my feet moving automatically beneath me, and do what comes naturally. I run.

When I finish, in 10 hours and 18 minutes, I'm overjoyed. Not because of my second-place finish among women—results always follow feeling—but because that day in the Caldera, I become an ultrarunner, a speck running through space, adrift between the enormity of earth and sky.

ADAPTED FROM "THE AGONY AND ECSTASY OF ULTRARUNNING" AND REPRINTED COURTESY OF OUTSIDE ONLINE.

TAKE IT *From* A MOTHER
WHERE IS THE MOST MEMORABLE PLACE YOU'VE RUN?

"Every year we camp in Zion National Park. My husband and I leave the kids with whichever mom comes with us, and we take the tram to the top of the canyon first thing in the morning. We run about 7 miles back to the campground. It's amazing to see the sunrise and the animals (wild turkeys, mule deer, condors). Best runs ever!"

—ALISSA (Favorite strength-training move: "Wait. You're supposed to strength train?")

"I ran 10 miles around a cruise ship track: 24 laps. For the first 12, I put a penny in a pile and then for the last 12, I picked up one of the pennies until there were none. Voila!"

—JESSICA (Forgot her Body Glide at a race, so used ChapStick under her bra.)

"My family ran the Freedom Trail 5K in Boston. It was the highlight of our vacation."

—ANGIE (Does squats by the back door while watching the sunrise and waiting for the dog to do his business.)

"I ran a spontaneous 5K on Disney's Castaway Cay in the Bahamas, my first race not on American soil. I had no idea they had an organized race. I had all my running stuff with me and said, 'Why not?'"

—KATHLEEN (Would like to run a marathon before she turns 50.)

Diego Garcia, which is in the Indian Ocean, seven degrees south of the equator. The island is thirty-seven miles from one tip to the other and only a few miles wide depending on the tide.

—KIM (Hardest place she's run? Afghanistan, where she was deployed. "The dust made it hard to breathe at times, and the rocks were determined to break my ankles.")

"I ran a race in Kelowna, B.C., called the Peak to Beak. It was 18K that went like this: down a mountain, along the lakefront, through the trails, and back up into a vineyard. Hard, cool, kinda exotic."

—KOURTNEY (Tried to streak—run 1 mile/day—for month of December. Made it eleven days. "Pitiful, I know.")

"By the Gulf of Mexico on South Padre Island. Running by the beach is the only time I don't need music."

—MOLLY (Pre-running, she had twenty-seven visual migraine headaches in a year. Post-running? Only two in past twenty-six months. "I no longer have to see a neurologist. Running has made a huge difference.")

"I love running in Rocky Mountain National Park. My favorite place on earth."

—LISA (Does school pick-up runs with the double jogger. The run there is with one kid and downhill, but going home—with two kids, backpack, lunch box, and a violin once—is mostly uphill.)

"I haven't done any exotic runs, but I will say running on a Florida beach at sunrise wasn't the dreamy experience I thought it would be. Running through sand is tough, and I discovered I'm more than a little afraid of crustaceans."

—STEPH (Sister-in-law told her to start her first marathon at the slowest pace she could imagine, and then slow it down even further. "I completely ignored this advice, flew through my first 16 miles, and bonked at 18. I'll be heeding her advice next marathon!"

"Doha, Qatar, where there was 80 percent humidity at 6 a.m. It was so hard to catch my breath. I thought I was having a pulmonary embolism from the thirteen-hour flight. Plus, I was not sure what I was allowed to wear and how much skin I could expose without being offensive to cultural norms. All that said, it's pretty neat to say I've run on the Persian Gulf."

—ROBIN (Has also run in -32° C [-25° F] wind chill, and gotten frostbite on both ears. "Once my husband reassured me my ears wouldn't fall off, I stopped whining a bit.")

Pre's Trail in Eugene, Oregon. I wasn't even dressed for it and it was raining—of course, it's Oregon!—but I loved every second of it. It felt like hallowed ground."

— KRISTEN (Gets down and planks regularly. "They work so much of what is important in running.")

COMING OF AGE
by Sarah Bowen Shea

Because it's mid-July here in Portland, sunlight sneaks through our bedroom blinds even though it's only 5:30 in the morning. I slowly open my often-creaky closet door in hopes of not waking my husband, Jack, or our light-sleeping, early rising son, John, whose bedroom is closest to ours. It's week five of training for the Victoria, B.C., marathon, and my coach has prescribed a 50-minute run with some *fartlek* speedwork sprinkled into the otherwise-comfortable running pace. Five bursts of 30-second intensity, then four repeats of 2 minutes of tempo effort. In an already challenging training plan that stretches out another three months, it's a four on a one-to-ten scale of tough.

I slip on a patterned running skirt just as Miller, our tabby cat, starts nudging my lower legs in hopes of getting fed. In one motion, I turn around and bend to pet him. When I stand back up, I'm greeted by my reflection in the full-length mirror on the back of the open closet door.

Slats of sunlight illuminate my save-for-the-skirt naked body. When, I wonder, did my barely B-cup breasts acquire the ability to hold a pencil under them? Even after breastfeeding all three of my children, my boobs had still held their own in the upright category. Now, I notice, they are melting down my ribs.

I rotate for a profile view. My stomach strains the skirt's waistband. My belly was always my least-favorite part of my 5' 11" body, but my loathing of it has only intensified since becoming a mother. After the birth of my older daughter, now twelve, I'd committed myself to twice-weekly Pilates classes. The Boat Poses, Hundreds, and other challenging, core-centric exercises finally had given my abs a wee bit of definition. For the first time since my early teens, I hadn't had to furiously suck in my gut at the pool.

Then I got pregnant with twins, and the duo did a number on those muscles, stretching them before they were sliced by the OB/GYN's scalpel. Despite now taking a barre-inspired class every Tuesday and Thursday, which serves up a fair share of strenuous ab work, I've lost hope of ever getting rid of my gut. Being launched into early menopause only made matters worse. As I stand gaping at my paunch, the term "menopot" springs to mind.

I slip a sports bra over my head to scoop up my heading-south chesticals, and numbers flitter through my mind. I've always had a good memory and a head for dates, which translates into being able to easily recall my race times. Plus, I work hard for my results, so I like having them handy in my back pocket to bolster my sports ego when it flags or, yes, to #humblebrag occasionally.

At age forty-three, I set all my big personal bests. A 1:46 half-marathon, 3:52 for the marathon, and equally speedy-for-me times in the 5K and 10K. Times that were, save for the half-marathon, the fastest in my life—not just that decade. I sigh, which only makes my bulging belly swell even more. I contemplate my current marathon goal—less than four hours—as I struggle to hook the bra's clasp. It was the number I strove for throughout my thirties, when I first started running 26.2-mile races.

My finish times of my previous ten marathons have mostly danced around the four-hour mark. A 4:03 in my debut marathon as a divorced-with-no-kids thirty-two-year-old. A 4:01 at age thirty-six, fourteen months after giving birth to our older daughter. The same time in the super-hilly Big Sur Marathon after training with a coach at age forty-four. A Boston-qualifying 3:59:54 later that same year.

After being sidelined with plantar fasciitis for roughly four months the next year, however, my times dramatically slowed down: 4:43 in the (record-hot) Boston Marathon and 4:08 in the Twin Cities 26.2. Going half the distance didn't help matters much: In the blink of an eye, it seemed, my half-marathon finish times all clustered around 1:58 or 1:59. No matter how hard I pushed over the course of the 13.1 miles, I barely squeaked in at less than two hours.

While my foot was hobbled with PF, my uterus had stepped out of line, deciding to bleed almost as often as it didn't. That summer was a sea of red that suddenly parted that autumn, leaving me without a period for almost a year. Just before I crossed the finish line into menopause (which is vaguely and frustratingly defined as the cessation of menstruation for twelve months), my period made a brief appearance, never to be seen again. I hadn't been hit hard with many menopausal symptoms like hot flashes or dry lady parts, but I didn't need an M.D. to connect the dots between menopause and tougher times, both physically and mentally, in races.

I was embarrassed to have gone into early menopause—psychologically, it made me feel like a senior citizen when it often seems like high school was years, not decades, ago. No one else needed to know I was now barren, but *I* knew, and I felt it as I hoofed around our neighborhood. Early menopause was like a banana peel I'd slipped on as I progressed along the aging-process path.

Even as I'm learning to cope with my menopot and all the other issues "The Change" brings, I have to acknowledge the main reason I'm slowing down: age. I could lose weight and regain some speed. (For every pound lost, studies suggest a runner can go two seconds faster per mile. Over the course of a marathon, losing five pounds would translate to finishing four minutes, twenty-two seconds faster; dropping ten pounds would shave almost nine minutes off the clock!) And I could redouble my effort at strengthening my core (recently, when I bemoaned my belly, Dimity suggested I hammer out a plank a day), and probably gain some seconds there. But I love desserts too much to drop any pounds and planking as I focus on my kids' candy wrappers under our basement couch just isn't going to happen. The hard truth is, like all us mother runners, I'm getting older. *Sigh.*

According to World Masters Athletics, runners slow about seven percent per decade in their forties, fifties, and sixties. (The decline is even more precipitous beyond that point.) In addition to having no head for science, I'm lousy at math, but good ol' Google tells me that means adding 4.2 minutes for every hour of race time for my golden 4:00 marathon. Right there, in one decade, is about 17 additional minutes. *Ouch.*

In my thirties and even early forties, any start-of-run sluggishness disappeared by the time my GPS beeped out the first mile. In my mid-forties, I needed to get 2 miles under my legs before they felt decent; now that I'm forty-eight, I feel slow and lumbering until mile 3. A 10:30- or 10:15-pace in those first few miles feels as strenuous as an 8:45 felt in my twenties or 9:15 felt in my thirties. It's demoralizing and daunting.

These days, once my engine gets moderately warm, it takes more effort to make it rev. My hips seem less willing to let my legs drive forward and back with sufficient intensity; my knees sometimes suddenly seem to zig when the rest of my body zags. (And now they *cr-cr-creak* whenever I squat to sit on the toilet.) If I stop too suddenly at an intersection, my glutes occasionally seize up. Even my stinking hammertoe—my curled-under, pork-rind of a right little toe—shrieks louder and more frequently during runs than it did even just a year ago.

For most of 2013, a year scattered with half-marathons but no 26.2s, I started to accept the fact I was almost a card-carrying AARP member. Running runDisney races made the I-am-getting-woefully-slower reality a bit easier to accept because those full-of-photo-ops races aren't about the time on the clock. I told myself my 2:15 at the 2013 Tinker Bell was because of posing with Mrs. Incredible and Aladdin, but when I was honest with myself, I admitted it was because I didn't have the juice to go faster.

Reluctant to stare down a start line knowing my finish time would only make me feel geriatric, not jaunty, I didn't race much in the spring and summer of 2013. Meanwhile, in "real" life, I kidded myself that the thatch of white hairs at my part blended in with my blonde highlights. As the months flew by, the furrow between my eyebrows became almost deep enough to plant a row of carrots.

As fall approached, a quick backwards-count on the calendar told my running partner, Molly, and me it was time to start training for our mid-January half-marathons. I was headed back to Disneyland for Tinker Bell, and Molly was running a small, tabletop-flat local race that promised fast times with diligent training. Despite my belief I no longer possess what it takes to fly, I jumped on a moderately aggressive training program to support Molly.

For the first time in more than a year, I put my nose to the workout grindstone. Tempo runs, intervals, and hill repeats. (I only remember where the big hills in our neighborhood are located because I'd been avoiding them for eighteen months!) My lungs heave, my quads ache, and my head feels a bit fuzzy after the bursts of exertion. But also I am exhilarated when Molly and I run 400-meter repeats at the recently refurbished high school track in 1:58s, then 1:55s, then 1:52s. We hit the track every Monday morning and do tempo runs every Wednesday. The more intense workouts restrict the flow of conversation, making me realize our runs over the past year had become in-motion gab sessions, not speed-honers.

One December morning, as heavy clouds obliterate the early morning light, Molly and I are running the second of two 2-mile tempo segments on a neighborhood street where the only inclines are speed bumps. We'd agreed we'd each run our own pace, and in the second mile, I am nearly two blocks ahead of Molly. My strides are relaxed and smooth, a gazelle-like sensation I hadn't felt in several years. At the end of the 2 miles, a smile creeps across my face between shallow, rapid breaths.

"You have newfound speed, Sarah," Molly pants. "You should run a race before Tinker Bell to see what you can really do."

For the next few days, Molly's comment bumps around in my brain. While I love running in a crowd of tutus, I needed fewer runners and cooler temps to know what I was capable of on a race course. With an abbreviated, four-day taper, I toe the start line of a holiday-themed half-marathon, replete with a green-and-red felt Christmas tree pinned to the back of my running vest. Surrounded by runners decked out in fuzzy reindeer antlers and candy-cane-striped knee socks, I am optimistic.

I give myself an unstructured time goal—closer to 1:50 than 1:55—to allow my pace to be fluid, rather than laser-beam precise. This race is about seeing what I have left in my legs, not fretting if varicose veins are developing on them. By mile 2, I surprise myself with how comfortable and controlled an 8:35 pace feels. I only occasionally glance at my GPS, choosing to run by perceived exertion; I'm aiming for a six or seven on a one-to-ten scale. I pay careful attention to fueling and hydration—Nuun and a GU at miles 4, 8, and 11—because gone are the days of winging it in a race.

The excitement of the crowd and seeing friends along the course carries me through mile 10. I dig a little deeper, and I spot runners to pass. My limbs feel surprisingly supple and cooperative, and I am able to maintain a brisk pace. In the final mile, the thrill of picking off runners, some of them firm of flesh and young of age, makes my steps feel a little lighter. Or maybe it's the slight downhill to the finish. Either way, my finish time is 1:53:12. Closer to 1:55 than I'd hoped, but an online search later tells me it's the fastest half-marathon I've run in more than three years. Meno-pot or no, my mother runner legs still have a spark.

Now, in the July morning light with Miller meowing insistently, I pull on my grey-and-pink Badass Mother Runner hat, and I stare at my reflection one final time. I know many challenging workouts—much closer to the "ten" end of the exertion scale than the "one" side—await me during the next few months of marathon prep. A sly smile creeps across my face. Sure, I have laugh lines and need reading glasses, but I also know with age comes wisdom. I am wise—and old—enough to know I have a few more good and speedy years left in this body.

TMI, THE EXTENDED EDITION

"So you're on a twelve-miler. You run out to the 6-mile turnaround, knowing full well you should've turned around at least a mile sooner. And then your lady business starts to shift, and you're 4 miles from home with your only tampon hanging out. You start thinking about knocking old guys off their bikes so you can steal them," writes Sadie, a mother runner with four kids. "This happens to everyone, right?"

Well, maybe not everyone, Sadie, but everyone has her version of TMI—too much information—at Another Mother Runner. Some are tame ("Sometimes I sweat a lot, and it looks like I peed," admits Sandra. "Really embarrassing."), and some are pretty intense. ("I suffered from a prolapsed bladder and a prolapsed rectum," writes Deb. "Yes, my rectum fell out of my vagina. Not pleasant to run with, let me tell you.") But there isn't any shortage of tales of leaky boobs, leaky bladders, and other "benefits" of being a mother runner.

If you haven't experienced the beauty of having blood streak your inner thigh as you streak home, you might consider this unnecessary potty talk. We beg to differ: Running isn't just about your lower limbs and your heart rate. Your whole body has to buy in, and when it doesn't, it's comforting to know you're not the only one in the boat, which just happens to have a little urine sloshing on the deck.

In case you don't believe us, here are some other TMI highlights:

"Since having my son, I have had bladder control problems: not leaking, but full-on wetting my pants. The worst time was at a 5K, when I was heading toward my PR and my personal goal of sub-30 minutes. After mile two, my bladder went, and every time I sped up after that, it happened more. I crossed the finish line with my PR, but not a sub-30 time, and I burst into tears."

—KERRIE (Happy ending: "I had a bladder sling placed a few months after that, and it was my best decision ever. I no longer wet my pants, even if I have coffee before a run.")

"On a long run, I was wearing a zip-front bra, and the zipper decided to come totally unzipped while I was on a lakefront path with people. It was really hard to get the zipper back together without looking like I was trying to flash everybody."

—ERIN (Was so paranoid about having her period on marathon race day, she thought about going on the Pill.)

"Never eat grapefruit the night before a long run. I crapped my way through 8 miles after doing so. Thankfully, it was early and I was at home on the treadmill. On the positive side, I was cleaned out like never before!"

—BEA (Her favorite Christmas present: subscription to *Runner's World*.)

"My period started the day before I was out for a point-to-point eighteen-miler. Somewhere around mile 13, I glanced down and realized the white trim on my sweat-soaked blue running shorts was, to my horror, red. The blood had mixed with the sweat and run down my legs and into my shoes. My laces were also red. I took my water bottles and sprayed down my legs and shorts as best I could."

—KATE (When she saw her family at the end, the first words out of her mouth, "Where are the keys? The truck? I need to get a towel around me.")

"My nose runs as fast as I do when I run, and I blow a ton of snot rockets. I imagine I'm invisible when I do it but once, during an especially productive post-cold rocket, a car pulled over and a woman offered me a tissue. Completely humiliating."

—MARY JO (Admits she's "avoided reaching out to a few women to go for a run out of fear it wouldn't go well and that it would make for awkward school exchanges going forward.")

"One long run, I wore my tight-fitting, super-cute purple shorts. Since they have a tiny liner in them, I did not wear panties—commando it is! I ran my 14 miles, free as could be, and it felt great. I get back home, finish sweating, and get in the shower. That is when I notice between my butt cheeks are *burning!* Just like when my upper arms chafe, but worse—because it was my b-u-t-t! For the rest of the day, I was very careful about sitting and standing, slowly."

—CHRISTINE (Runs to a mix of her teen's pop music and husband's Texas country because she's too busy running to download her own tunes.)

"While on a trail run, I stood to pee. I ran off of the trail, pulled the shorts of my running skirt over to the side, took a wider stance, pushed really hard with my abdominal muscles, and went. It's a lot less messy than squatting and having pee land in my shoes. I revealed this secret to my husband years later, and he stared at me blankly and said, 'Don't tell me things like that.'"

—LISA (Frequently followed by a Lab on her runs, even though he is not her dog. Maybe he wants to mark his territory, too?)

"When I started getting bikini line chafing on my long runs, I figured it was time to tame my high-tensile-strength pubes with a wax. Everyone said waxing was more effective and hygienic than shaving. Being a do-it-yourself kind of gal, I bought the best wax and prepared to wince, though I was looking forward to baby-smooth skin under my shorts. Imagine my dismay when the result, a day before my long run, was only partial success and a swath of angry, red bumps that lingered for days and resulted in numerous ingrown hairs. My trusty razor and I have never looked back!"

—ANG (Loves half-moon pose in yoga. "Standing poses really work all your leg muscles, big and small.")

"Five a.m. run along a river trail, when I had to go number two. I searched for the nearest grove of trees or bushes and spotted the only option. I squatted to do my business. Suddenly, I was attacked by a mama goose that chose this very same secluded spot to make her nest! She went totally nuts on me while I was in a very compromising position. Goose bites hurt!"

—LIESA (Told people she was "pregnant, but not broken" when they commented on her running preggo.)

"I ran the Warrior Dash and forgot to remove the Poise pad I wear daily for pee leaks. During the swimming portion, the pad ballooned inside my shorts. I looked like I dropped a load in my shorts. I had to duck behind a tree and remove the nastiness without anyone seeing me."

—LASHELL (Favorite sports bra: "whatever is on clearance at Target.")

"After the birth of my daughter, I didn't experience any leakage problems while running until I came back to coach high school cross-country. Then I discovered I can run *or* I can shout, but I can't do both at the same time."

—ELIZABETH (Also discovered "it's important to keep your cool around teenagers so they don't realize you've peed your shorts.")

"My husband, who doesn't 'get' my running, works from home. After an incredibly long run, I hit the shower. I hear the bathroom door open, and I figure it's my young daughter since we share a bathroom. Nope. The shower curtain slides back, and my dear hubby slides into the shower with me. The last thing I'm going to say is, 'Sorry, honey, I just went running.' I would hereby like to nominate my husband for the 'World's Worst Timing' award."

—HEATHER (Not afraid to stop mid-run to take photos of venomous snakes.)

"When I ran the Buffalo Marathon, I disregarded everything I know about prerace fueling and ate a veggie burger, big salad, and corn on the cob for dinner the night before. Sisters, let me tell you: If you choose to follow this fueling plan, you will stop in six porta-potties, and you will live to see that whole cornucopia of fiber come back to haunt you."

—MEG (Mantra: "Let your legs fall free and easy; let your body be loose and light.")

"Had the big O once during a run. Maybe it's the way the tights were rubbing?"

—STACY (When questionable-looking person is approaching her on a run, she "mentally reviews my Krav Maga lessons.")

"After having children, I get an occasional flair-up of hemorrhoids from strenuous activity. I'm training for my fifth marathon and, wouldn't you know it, the 'roids are back and worse than ever. I've taken time off from exercise, tried over-the-counter remedies, and even seen the doctor, who told me to just give it time. I'm so desperate to relieve the size, I even tried doing yoga postures, including headstands."

—LIZ (Started running one-milers with her own marathon mom at age six.)

"Because of some explosive GI issues, I had to squat in a wheat field once. While I was doing my business, a tractor came tooling down the gravel road right by me. And one of my husband's coworkers was driving the tractor. I hid in the wheat, and to this day, don't know if he saw me or not."

—JESSICA (Wants to run the Marine Corps Marathon. "I get to run a marathon, then my family can enjoy DC together.")

"Chafing on the girl parts. Ouch!"

—MOLLY (Dream race: Boston Marathon. "Just eight minutes faster to qualify!")

"On pit stops in Mother Nature, I got poison ivy where the sun doesn't shine. Not once, but twice!"

—JOAN (Hates running injuries. "Why is that people who are trying to be healthy and active get sidelined?")

"Immodium is a must for me. I have to take one the night before any race, even a 5K, or I would sit forever on the toilet the following morning. Also, I had a cup of coffee before my first half-marathon to warm up. Never again."

—LARAE (When she lost a toenail, she bragged about it.)

"Oh, geez. My first half-marathon last fall was during my period. I wore a tampon, and by mile 9 the flow was so heavy my tampon was coming out! I pulled off into the woods, reached into my shorts to pull it out, and wrapped it in a Kleenex I was carrying. There was a restroom about a mile ahead, and it could not have come fast enough!"

—TRISH (Geeks out on old *Star Trek* episodes on the treadmill.)

"I have two tubes of Body Glide: one for my body, and the other clearly, boldly, marked, 'ASS.' When it comes time to lube up before a run, I do *not* want to confuse those two!"

—AMY (Careful readers will recognize this is a repeat from *Train Like a Mother*, but it's SBS's all-time fave, so we brought it back.)

07

PERSISTENCE:
Hang on; You've Got This

"Running and I are like a dysfunctional couple. It's good for me; I'm not good at it. It hurts me, I love it. I ignore it, it hurts me worse. It makes me hot, but my mom is convinced it'll break my leg. We drift apart, I start again. Every few months, we're perfectly in sync. It's those good times that keep me going."

—MEGAN

IF YOU DON'T RUN, YOU CAN'T WIN
by Terzah Becker

My six-year-old son, Will, discovered detective stories last year and decided he wanted to be a private eye himself. His business plan was simple: He'd tape several signs advertising his services to the front window of our house (example: WILL BECKER DETECTIV $1 SOVS MISTREES), and hang out in the front yard. He figured he'd be soving mistrees in no time.

Except—no surprise—it didn't work. He got no clients.

"Will," I said, "you didn't give it enough time. Starting a business is hard work!"

I hoped I sounded wise to him, but maybe I was just annoying. Either way, Will comes honestly by his impatience and his desire for things to be easy. He is my child, after all. I started running way back in 1985, when I was twelve, because adolescence made me suddenly pudgy and I didn't like that. I didn't like running much at first, either. I did it only for weight-maintenance benefits until I entered a 10K as an adult on a whim. I discovered I actually liked racing even though it was clear I wasn't going to break records. I finished my first marathon two years later on an unusually cold day in Houston. It took me five hours. I didn't think I needed or wanted to do another one, ever.

But somewhere between leaving a grueling newspaper job to join the Peace Corps and meeting my husband, Dan, I changed my mind. The year we got married, I trained for and ran the New York City Marathon. My time was faster than it had been eight years earlier: 4:14. Fairly content, I shelved marathons for a while because I got pregnant with Will and his twin sister, Ruthie. As I was training for New York, though, I had heard about the Boston Marathon and wondered if I could do that. The question lingered as my kids grew from babies into toddlers and I found more time for running again.

The Boston Marathon. It's basically the one 26.2 in the U.S. that you can't just pay for and cross the finish line. You have to run a prior marathon at a challenging-for-most-of-us pace and finish under a certain time, which qualifies you to enter. (Hence the acronym BQ: Boston Qualifier). The finishing time is based on your age and gender. For me at age thirty-seven, nestled in the thirty-five-to-thirty-nine age group, I needed to run a 3:45 or faster. (There is an exception for runners who raise a lot of money for charity. As difficult—and noble—as doing that is, I wanted to be a BQ. I'd heard it's something only ten percent of all marathoners can accomplish, and that quest appealed to me the way getting into prestigious universities had when I was a junior in high school.)

I thought my fortieth birthday, then a little more than two years away, would be a reasonable and nicely symbolic deadline for the goal. I also thought it would give me a cushion, one I hoped I wouldn't need. Each jump forward in an age group nets 5 more qualifying minutes, so I could potentially "just" have to run 3:50. I didn't tape a sign to my front window that said SLOWER RUNNER WANTS TO RUN BOSTON. PLEASE GIVE THAT TO ME. But I wanted to do this hard thing without it being hard.

That fall, there were a lot of objective strikes against me. My best marathon time was still that 4:14 from NYC, nearly a half-hour slower than 3:45—and I'd run that race before Will and Ruthie brought all the changes having kids bring to your body and schedule. Also, the year had been tough on my whole household in terms of illnesses and lost sleep. The twins, now three, had started preschool and brought home one cold after another, along with strep throat and pneumonia, and caring for them at night compounded the effects of the insomnia I'd dealt with since they were born. I was weak in both body and mind.

To top it off, a couple of months after I started training, Boston Marathon officials decided to make all the qualifying times stricter. Not only did they make them faster by five minutes, they eliminated the 59-second cushion they previously had allowed. A 3:45:59 would've got me in before; now I definitely needed sub-3:45:00, and ideally, a sub-3:40:00, if I wanted a true BQ by the time I turned forty. (Nerdy rule reader here: You can BQ at age thirty-nine with a sub-3:45, provided you'll be forty on the day you race Boston.)

Despite my public acknowledgment of those obstacles—I paid a lot of lip service to the fact I had to improve my time by 30 minutes and was trying to work thirty hours a week as a librarian and raise young twins at the same time—my private attitude was like Will's toward becoming a detective: I *wanted* to qualify and therefore I figured I *would*. I thought showing up for the training would do it. I've always been good at showing up, at doing everything in my assignment notebook on schedule and to the letter. But Boston isn't algebra, and just showing up wasn't going to cut it.

My first two attempts at BQ were encouraging. I started with the Top of Utah Marathon. The course runs down a beautiful canyon for the first 15 miles, and I foolishly—but understandably— got carried away by the stunning surroundings and all that luscious downhill. The 8:20/mile pace I ran for some of those early miles meant that when I hit mile 16 and flat ground, I smashed into a wall as thick as those of the canyon I just floated down. I ended up walking much of the last part. Still, I squeaked under four hours for a near-15-minute personal record.

Four months later, just before my thirty-ninth birthday, I headed south to run the Houston Marathon, site of my first effort at 26.2 fifteen years prior. Bearing in mind what had happened in Utah, I eased into the race. My first mile was my slowest—the speed-up-slowly-through-the-race strategy most experts recommend—and I shaved my PR down to 3:53, feeling strong the whole way. Though still far from 3:45 and very far from 3:40, it was steady progress. I secretly thought I'd nail the sub-3:45 in the fall, comfortably before my fortieth birthday.

That simple progression, though, was not to be. Just two weeks after Houston, a back issue stemming from a weak core relegated me to the recumbent bike for four months. I was nervous, but still believed I could nab BQ that year. Not taking any chances, I hired an excellent local coach, Darren De Reuck, who also coaches his wife, Olympic marathoner Colleen De Reuck. With professional advice and workouts, I seemed to be on the comeback trail. In front of friends and Dan, I ran the Detroit Half-Marathon in 1:47, a 10-minute PR and a strong indicator I had the fitness to beat 3:45 at my next marathon.

But Detroit was my only bright spot for a full twelve months. My final 26.2 as a thirty-nine-year-old was the California International Marathon in December 2012, a race now infamous for its headwinds and torrents of rain. I knew the forecast going into it, but nonetheless when I crossed the line in 4:06, I felt utterly downcast, like a loser.

I blew out forty candles on my birthday cake and pushed on past the blown deadline, only to suffer another defeat. At my seventh marathon and fourth BQ attempt, the Eugene Marathon in Oregon, I let the emotion of the Boston bombings get to me and once again went out too fast, slowed way down after mile 17, and death-marched it in for a 3:57. I'm not a big crier, but I wept in that finishers' area next to storied Hayward Field, with my two best running friends, Cynthia and Kathy, patting me on the back. After that race, I ran two lousy half-marathons. I wondered if the BQ really was too hard for me. Maybe, I thought, I should end the quest and try to be happy with my PRs.

Somehow, though, amid all that failure, something in me changed. I wanted to keep at it. I wanted to prove my race in Detroit wasn't a fluke, that all the time and money I'd spent for more than three years hadn't been wasted. So instead of quitting, I shrugged off the recent defeats. I went online and found stories of other runners who'd had a long road but finally made it to Boston. I adopted a new motto, a line from *Chariots of Fire*: "If you don't run, you can't win." I put the Chicago Marathon on the calendar. I would try again.

As the training for Chicago unfolded, I took an honest look at my biggest weakness: not embracing the discomfort a BQ required. I needed to learn to hurt, to realize that hurting doesn't mean a race is over. So I ran in hot weather (which I hate), bore down in speed workouts, went to bed and got up early, and didn't shy away from hills and faster-than-comfortable paces in my weekend long runs. I remember one workout in particular. On a hot August Saturday, I got up at 4:30 a.m. and ran 10 miles to meet up with Colleen De Reuck's running club, the Boulder Striders, for a hard workout on a hilly, dusty trail. And I nailed it, notching 20 miles total by the time Dan and the kids arrived to pick me up. I also paid more attention to my diet, avoiding sweets and drinking a daily V8 to make up for a lack of creativity with vegetables. I occasionally lapsed into fantasy. As my speedwork started getting speedier, I envisioned myself crossing the line in Chicago under a clock that read 3:38, a highly unlikely number even with newfound swiftness. Mostly, though, I concentrated on the workout for the day and forced myself to take the attitude that a well-executed race and a personal record would be enough in Chicago, with or without a BQ.

The morning of October 13 dawned chilly and clear in Chicago. My strategy: to stick with the 3:45 pacer "like a fly on his back," per Darren's instructions. Given my near-perfect training that summer, I thought Darren was being conservative, but staying just below the required 8:34/mile pace—which the pacer was holding—proved hard from the start. It had been a while since I had run a big-city race like this one, and the sheer number of runners clustering around the three pacers meant sticking to them like a pesky insect wasn't easy. I felt out of control. The noisy crowds in the first couple of miles spooked me, too. I didn't talk to anyone, but I did notice a couple of other women around my age with determined looks; I clearly wasn't the only forty-something out there for the BQ. Seventeen miles in, about where I'd bonked in Eugene, I was still with the pacers, though still not feeling as great as I'd have liked. I kept wanting to slow down because the effort didn't feel easy.

Around mile 20, I stopped and, to avoid bending over, asked a spectator to tie my shoe and saw those pacers receding in the distance. I realized how deep my desire was to do it this time. My nice shoe-tie guy asked if I wanted a double knot. Not wanting to waste another second, I said, "No thanks!" and took off. I ran steady, caught the pacers with a couple of 8:20 miles and passed them to finish in 3:44:06.

I had done it. It wasn't a BQ by the triumphant margin I'd envisioned in my wilder dreams, but it was the real thing and a 9-minute PR to boot. Swathed in my space blanket, I high-fived race volunteers. I laughed out loud. I called Dan and Kathy and Cynthia. I sent Darren the results and was thrilled when he told me, almost casually, that we'd get a 3:40 next.

Three tough years of striving had taught me lessons I needed to learn: patience, perseverance, humility. I realized I can accomplish hard things, but doing so means doing more than the equivalent of hanging up a sign saying "I want to . . ." then waiting for it to happen. Sometimes simply not quitting in the face of disappointment is the most important (and hardest) part. I hope my kids learn that lesson sooner than I did.

There's hope for that, too. When I came home from Chicago, Ruthie had made a sign depicting a stick-figure me leaping over a mountain. Will, who has moved on from detectives and now wants to be Harry Potter, had made one that said: MOM KWALIFYED FOR BOSTON. MOM WON!

I didn't correct them. I've never worked so hard or long for anything. I did, in fact, win.

TAKE IT *From* A MOTHER
WHAT IS THE MOST CHALLENGING ASPECT OF RUNNING FOR YOU?

"Finding time and energy. It's not easy to get on the treadmill at 9 p.m. after working all day and chasing a toddler all evening."

—MARY (Used a real-estate flyer from a FOR SALE sign to blow her nose, mid-run.)

"Allowing myself to take it easy."

—LAUREN (Founder of the annual "Lauren Maleski I'm Too Cheap to Pay for a Half-Marathon Half-Marathon.")

"Running wisely enough to avoid injury."

—STACEY (Her Road ID reads: "Stacey, if you can walk it—you can run it.")

"Getting back on board after a hiatus like injury or pregnancy. It's hard to respect where I am now, without comparing my speed/body/endurance to a previous best."

—MEG (After reading that smiling and positive self-talk can positively influence your exertion, she says hello to every pedestrian she passes. "Even the grumps.")

"Getting over my own head games. I can run a marathon with confidence, and two weeks later, be nervous about an easy four-miler."

—JILLIAN (During her first 5K, she ran with her husband, who pushed the double stroller. "I made him promise not to step over the finish line before me. I couldn't believe I had run 3 straight miles!"

"Running farther than 9 miles."

—KELLSEY (That said, always considered herself a ten-minute-miler, but "Turns out I can run 13.1 miles at a 9:41 pace. Who knew?")

"That my knees and feet are ready to stop way before my mind, heart, or lungs are."

—AMY (Describes her running as "slow, but progressing.")

"Speedwork. I know I need to do it to improve, but it's never easy."

—LISA (Q: What's the strongest part of your body? A: "My quads." Q: How'd they get that way? A: "Running, silly.")

*"The last 6 miles of a marathon, when my brain says
'hell no' and my legs listen . . . and I give in."*

—MANDY (She urged five of her coworkers to run a half-marathon with her. "They
all did it! I cried and cheered for each one of them when they finished.")

*"Being a bigger runner. I wasn't skinny before kids, and I am not skinny now.
I started running for weight control, but now it's so much more than that. I
do find it hard when I am running with a bunch of cute skinny mamas, then
I realize they have the same stretch marks and determination I do."*

—MELISSA (Advice for avoiding shin splints: "When your shins feel like
they're pulling your muscles off, listen and chill out.")

*"Finding new routes. I could tell you the distance to everything within
10 miles of my house. I'm limited by which directions I can run. I can't
cross the expressway, and I'm surrounded by water on one side."*

—JILL (Her "ass crack" has chafed during races. "Kind of hard to lube with
Body Glide, and Vaseline just feels all kinds of wrong.")

*"I run at 5 a.m., but getting up early is not the challenge.
Shutting off my brain—and the computer—and going to bed
early and keeping my husband happy . . . all challenges."*

—JAMIE (Doesn't mind doing 18- to 20-mile runs solo.
"I like to know I can gut it out even when I don't have anyone to distract me.")

*"Not letting the time for running slip away when I am not training for a
race. It gets too easy to give up my 'me time' for time with my kids."*

—MELISSA (Her two ten-pound-plus babies "crushed my abs. They've never been able to meet in the middle again.")

"Remembering my race photos are not a true representation of my running ability!"

—DEB (Race outfit rule: Always wear pink.)

3.1 MILES: TAKING CONTROL OF ME
by Amy Bailey

I'm watching DVR'd episodes of *The Biggest Loser* from the treadmill in my basement. Not surprisingly, Jillian Michaels is barking "Go faster!" at the sister team of Olivia and Hannah, but in my mind, she's yelling at me. The treadmill display blares 6.3 miles per hour, a 9:22 mile. Which is slower than the 8:59 mile (or 6.7 mph that I want be going) in my self-titled Amy's Fast 5K. But I don't know if I can handle pushing the up arrow on the speed another four times to reach the exertion my brain considers legitimately fast. My legs are sore, and the side of my neck is screaming, and with good reason: I raced in a half-marathon two days ago.

Above me, the house is dark. (It's always dark before 6 a.m. in northeast Wisconsin.) My three-year-old son and my husband are still sleeping. I've already let out my Corgi-mix dog, Franklin, without making eye contact with him so I don't feel guilty about the *please-walk-me-lady* look he always gives me. The only thing on this early, early morning agenda: speed through a 5K.

Around me, on the otherwise nondescript walls, is a corkboard with my bibs and other running mementos. The elegant medal—it's got shades of Tiffany blue and a black ribbon—from the 2011 Fueled by Fine Wine Half-Marathon, held in Oregon's Willamette Valley, hangs prominently in front of my other medals. It was that medal that spawned Amy's Fast 5K, now a ritual after every half-marathon.

After running the Big Sur Half-Marathon in the fall of 2010, I kept up my weekly mileage to make sure I would be ready for the hilly, treacherous course when I returned to the West Coast six months later. Long run after long run included a massive bridge and some rolling hills on a nearby college campus. I cranked up the incline on the treadmill. I was ready.

Despite all the vertical I ran in Wisconsin, though, I managed to rack up a PW (personal worst) in Oregon. The never-ending hills through the pinot noir-producing vines felt like mountains to this flatlander. "I just want to run for a continuous mile," I gasped to my sister as we climbed, descended, pounded over tough trails as clay dust ballooned under our feet, then climbed and descended some more. "That's it: just one straight mile."

I don't think I did get in a straight-up mile. I finished in 2:30:37, 20 to 30 frustrating, heartbreaking minutes slower than most of my half-marathon times. The finish line didn't hold its usual feelings of accomplishment and relief. Instead, I felt let down and pissed off. Part of me wanted to yell at the race organizers, "Why would you design a course like that?"

When I finally got to my car at the Green Bay airport, my thoughts moved ahead to the following day. I knew I needed to get over the race that literally sucked the wind out of me. I immediately thought of the treadmill in my basement. I wanted to feel the opposite of race day. I wanted fast, not a slow slog; I wanted flat, not impossible hills; I wanted to feel powerful, not empty; I wanted to race, not just cover ground.

I wanted to run Amy's Fast 5K.

Amy's Fast 5K has become as important as taking an extra-long shower after a race. Some might call it OCD to blitz through a 5K within days of covering 13.1 miles, but I call it TCOM: Taking Control of Me. Through 3.1 miles, I quiet the thing that scares me most about training for a race and crossing a finish line: what happens afterward. Through 3.1 miles, I reassure myself I'm in control of the after—and myself.

Beer, buffalo wings, onion rings, and Sunday-afternoon football. And cigarettes. There were a lot of those things in the years after my wedding in 2002. What there wasn't much of was the hardcore workout mentality that got me down to record-low weight when I walked down the aisle in a record-low-size white dress. A few months after the big day, I cancelled the gym membership to "save money" and told myself over and over that, "Why yes, walking the dog around the block every other day is exactly the same as a half hour on an elliptical!"

I walked away from fitness, but I was always, *always* captivated by running. I loved watching runners, and I wanted to be one of them so badly. In a New Year's Eve haze at the end of 2004, I resolved to run a 5K the following year. It never happened. It wasn't until three years later—and three moves and a baby in my belly—that we purchased a treadmill. With my already hot-and-cold attitude about going to the gym *and* a baby on the way, I knew a treadmill in the house was going to be the only way that regular workouts would happen. Still, I didn't really start running until the baby was nine months old.

When I finally got on it, the miles made me feel like the old Amy, the girl who played volleyball and softball in high school. Not like the current nicotine-addicted, trans-fat-loving Amy, the one who would get super-psyched about working out and then go days—and sometimes months—selectively forgetting the same workout bag stayed tucked in the backseat of her car.

After finally realizing that time to work out wouldn't just suddenly show up, I did what so many other mother runners do: I bit the bullet and set the alarm clock super-early. I won't lie: Getting up early is hard and it takes time to not hate it, but I finally feel ownership of that predawn time, when my temples pour sweat. To be able to thrive when most of Wisconsin isn't even up requires much more than the swipe of a finger to select an alarm. It means being prepared. I had to go into every workout with a plan, a training regime that would tell me exactly what I had to do.

Once I picked a plan, I just did it. I put myself on autopilot and got up to do what the plan told me to do. Three tempo miles on Monday, six at race pace on Thursday. Then, week after week, the "Can I really run *that* far?" long run on Saturday. My days were filled with decisions on everything from the basic ("Is today's cafeteria offering healthy enough to give into the child's pleas for a hot lunch?") to the more complex ("How do I tell my kid to *not* be a tattletale?"). It was a relief to have something that just says two miles of hill repeats. I could do that.

Problem is, every training plan eventually ends. Regular Tuesday tempo runs are replaced by a blank slate and anxiety. One question always bobs around in my head: Will I go back to being the sedentary, pudgy, not-really-happy person I used to be? Will I keep the basement door shut so I don't even catch a whiff of the treadmill? Will I milk the 1,500 calories I just burned during the half-marathon and eat or drink anything I want for a week—or, let's be honest, a month? Nope, I TCOM. I focus my vision straight ahead. I dial into the possibilities of tomorrow. Instead of chalking up the week—or even the month—to a lost cause because of a missed workout or the caloric onslaught of a four-course meal, I think about the comeback. The Fast 5K.

Five years into crossing plenty of finish lines, I know running isn't just about calorie burning, and banishing my buffalo-wing lifestyle. Running is a part of me and part of my day. I love the feeling of exhausted legs and tight arms so much more than a cold beer. (But let's be honest: I kind of love them both.) Running gives me time to think, time to look around, and most importantly, time to be prepared for the day that lies ahead. As I have increased my weekly mileage, my daily cries at work have almost disappeared. The periodic feelings of being overwhelmed are still there, but they're manageable. Because of running.

I'm 2.4 miles into the seventh time I've run Amy's Fast 5K. I'm going faster than two days ago because I can. Because I get to. And because somewhere way back in my past, I didn't think I could. And I want to keep that past exactly where it belongs: in a place it can't ever catch me again.

Below me, the treadmill belt is whirring and my legs are pounding the metal frame. My legs are relatively loose. I'm shaking out my arms every half-mile; they help me drive this running bus. I find motivation in those arm strokes, those regular pumps that push my hands into my field of vision. I'm watching another season of *The Biggest Loser* on the TV in our newly finished basement, but I can barely even hear Jillian. My mind is on the treadmill's distance counter. I promised myself I'd crank it up from 6.6 to 6.7 at the next mile marker and . . . it's . . . almost . . . here.

TAKE IT *From* A MOTHER
HOW OFTEN DO YOU THINK ABOUT QUITTING*?

that specific run/race—not the sport altogether

"Not often—and not until I'm close enough to get home or to the car easily. The exception: unless I feel injured/real pain/about to poop my pants—then I walk home or call my husband for a ride STAT."

—CAROLYN (Used running to get over severe depression. "I'd get out and run because changing my physiology seemed to change my emotions, if only for the day.")

"Never during an easy run, but I hate tempo runs. During those, I have to constantly tell myself to keep going."

— RENEE (Biggest complaint about running, besides tempo runs: "Running clothes are expensive!")

"During my marathons, I have spent miles 16 to 20 thinking about how wonderful half-marathons are, and how I should really stick to those."

—CARA (Met her best running friend, Patty, on a trail. "We spent a few weeks running by each other before Patty introduced herself and asked if I wanted to run with her.")

"Rarely, but I think about walk breaks all the time. I have only bailed on two runs, when plantar fasciitis was building."

—NIKKI (Doesn't know how much weight she's lost through running, but catches herself checking out her butt in the bathroom mirror. "So that must be a good sign.")

"Pretty much the whole time I'm running. While training for a half-marathon, I'd ask my friend, 'Whose bright idea was this?'"

—ANDREA (It was her bright idea.)

"On the treadmill, usually at least once. Or if my daughter is upstairs throwing a fit, I feel like quitting, but I remember her dad is perfectly capable of handling the issue. When I hear both of them throwing a fit, I really want to quit."

—TIFFANY (Description of her running: "Slow. Long. Yay.")

"Not even in my vocabulary. Not because it's always easy and not because I don't have runs I wish were over sooner, but because I don't consider it an option to quit. The disappointment I would feel in my self would not be worth the instant gratification of taking the easy way out."

—JODI (Her motto, cribbed from her six-year-old when she took on the monkey bars for the first time: "Just believe you can do it.")

"Two to three times in the first mile, but it goes away after that."

—JESSICA (Has to run until she hits her target mileage. "6.1 miles is okay, 5.9 is not.")

"Only when my body tells me I need to quit—then I listen and cut the run short. Mentally, I'm always good."

—ANNA (Worked up to running a mile by adding a mailbox each run.)

"It really depends. Sometimes I think about it the whole time, especially if I'm on the treadmill. Sometimes I get lost in my thoughts or music and feel like I could go forever. Those awesome runs are why I keep lacing up."

—MAIJA (Considers running with pepper spray since she's had a few close calls with unfriendly dogs.)

"For the whole first half of the run—no matter how far I am going—I think about it about once every minute or so. Once I've got past halfway, I generally stop being so obsessed, and think about it, say, only once every five minutes!"

—CLAIRE (Loves half-marathons. "Long enough that people are impressed— shallow, me?—but not so long that training runs dominate the weekends.")

"Never. I need to get back to where I started to get that coffee!"

—RUTH (Wants to run the Nike Women's Marathon for the finishers' necklace from Tiffany. "Only way I'll ever get one from there.")

"Once I get out the door, it's more of a 'Do I have to go back now?'"

— CARRIE (Hits the sweet spot about 16 minutes into a run.)

NINE RUNS, NINE LIVES
by Rachel Walker

1. *"Cross-country for me is the truest sport."*

I am sixteen years old and standing in front of my cross-country team at our high school's end-of-season banquet. My hands shake as I grip my spiral-bound journal. I asked for this pulpit, but right now I regret it and wonder why my coaches said yes. Out of pity, maybe. I suspect that's why they recruited me to the team in the first place.

"Team sports, such as soccer and basketball, are simply games with a winner and a loser. In cross-country, there is always a winner, but there are no losers. Granted, someone comes in last, but that person hasn't lost."

I am a scrappy runner, dogged in my pursuit of the girls ahead of me on the varsity roster. My goals are twofold: to lose weight and to gain a place in the world, a platform independent of my home, and of my mom and my stepdad and the tension between them, a fraught anxiety fueled by vodka and denial.

"Running has helped teach me it is not in my successes that I should look for praise but in my strivings. It has also taught me I don't need to look for affirmation from other people; I will find it in myself."

What I don't write or say: Running cross-country put an end to my fledgling eating disorder, and it's the reason I stopped filching smokes from my stepdad's packs. Because of my teammates, who are as studious as they are sinewy, I worked harder and took pride in my good grades.

"I love the sweat and pain of running hard. I love feeling winded and wobbly after an incredibly hard workout. I know if I want to reach a certain time and if I want it badly enough and work hard and relax enough, someday I'll achieve it."

When I'm done, one of my coaches asks me to type up the entire transcript. He sends it into *Runner's World,* and it will be published in the fall 1993 issue, my first step toward a career as a professional writer.

I don't know then it will take years to appreciate the wisdom of my teenage author self.

All I know is I've discovered running, and it will change the course of my life.

2. I've talked my way into a run on a steep trail in Vermont's Green Mountains. Two nice guys from my freshman art class at Middlebury College said I could tag along. I thought I'd feel at home. Instead, the root-choked, slippery trails are as foreign to this Colorado girl as the prep-school cul-

ture of my new, tiny, liberal arts world. I grunt up the trail, determined to prove my strength to the boys, whose enviable ease keeps the conversation light and airy.

At the summit, we guzzle water and then the boys spring away like puppies. I begin the descent on a slick path that plummets straight down, switchbacks be damned. When I catch a toe and stumble, momentum propels me onto a granite boulder and then into a thicket of tangled branches, shrubs, and stumps. Something pierces the skin around my knees and elbows. The boys, too far ahead, don't hear me. I walk the remaining 3 miles, blood streaming down my limbs.

When I reach them at the trailhead, they look me up and down, fail to register my stifled sobs, and exclaim, "Cool! Blood."

I know then I'll choose to run alone for now. And that's enough to take away the sting, if not the mess.

3. For my junior year abroad, I traveled halfway around the world to Madagascar. After three months of organized classes, my group was set free with the mandate to complete an independent-study project during the remaining month of the semester. I chose to explore the myths, traditions, and beliefs surrounding childbirth, which is how I found myself sitting inside a one-room hut deep in the rainforest with a Malagasy midwife and my translator. The old midwife stood five feet tall with a wrinkled-apple face, bright eyes, and two thick braids. I sat on a straw mat on the dirt floor while a fire burned in the hearth and smoke charred the wooden walls.

"Ask her what she does if the mother is scared when she's giving birth," I said to my translator.

The midwife cocked her head and gave me a puzzled look.

"She doesn't understand," my translator said.

"If the mother's nervous, how does she comfort her? Does she do something special to put the birthing mother at ease?"

The midwife lunged forward and exclaimed, "No!" She grabbed my knees and forced them apart. Her face rushed in front of mine, and her open mouth flapped with noise. She pried my legs even wider, and then slid her hands from my knees to my ankles. Her eyes bored into mine, and through the translator, she said, "This is what I do if the mother is scared. I hold her like this, and I bring her baby into the world."

My skin radiated with the heat of her hands when she finally peeled herself away, and I fought the urge, desperate and visceral, to spring from her hut and run as fast and hard as I could out of the forest, out of the towns, out of the country.

All I wanted in that moment was to run home.

4. At 23, I cannot relate to Pam's fear of a loveless and childless future. She's twelve years my senior, and her married boyfriend broke up with her last night. She called this morning in tears, and I arrived an hour later with a bottle of sparkling wine, orange juice, and chocolate croissants, which we consumed in quick order. The rich and alcoholic combination sunk her mood even deeper. "Cheer up," I offer. "He's a jerk. You're better off without him." I'm bright with optimism, certain of the benevolence of the universe. She shakes her head and says I don't understand. She's in her mid-thirties. She wants a baby. She loved him.

I don't buy it. My life has just begun. To me, the difference in our ages means nothing. Pam and I are two mountain women, united in solidarity. Her boyfriend was a jerk, a married-to-some-one-else jerk. She's better off without him. Enough talk. I've brought my running clothes, and I tell her to go change. We head out fifteen minutes later, and I take up the rear as we follow a trail through aspen groves. I wish Pam could see what I see: a beautiful and strong woman who deserves an honest man. We crest a hill, and she stops, doubling over with effort, complaining about fatigue, saying she's going to walk. "No, not an option," I say. I gently put my hand on the small of her back and guide her forward. At first she resists, then she relaxes and relents. Her body stretches, and her feet pound the dirt in rhythm. I follow, and soon we're running in sync. Our lives might be disparate, but right now on this run, we are on common ground.

5. Overnight the world has turned to ice. This is not the Oregon I know, and I walk outside disoriented. The ground creaks, and the dry, freezing air hurts my lungs. The sun starts to rise as I make my way toward central Oregon's Deschutes River. The cold slips through an opening between my top and tights and burns my skin. At the dike I realize the trails are impassable because of the ice.

I should have stayed in bed, which is not what I really wanted. I wanted a hard, sweaty workout in the same desperate way I wanted Bend to feel like home. Bend, where the people are nice and look like they should be my friends. We're all sporty. Skiers. Runners. Subaru drivers. But everyone I meet has come to this rising star of a town with someone else—a husband, a partner. They're building a life, and I'm just passing through.

I'm about to give in to the loneliness and head home when a herd of deer emerges from a stand of pine trees ahead. They startle when they see me and scatter. I'm frozen by their grace, the way they appear to float above the surface without crashing through. *Bounce! Bounce! Bounce!* I say the words quietly, my breath alighting in steamy frost as soon as it hits the chilly air. The deer disappear into the landscape, barely leaving footprints.

I begin to run once more, and this time my legs move on their own, strong and willing. I run in the direction of where the deer were, gaining momentum, gaining lightness. I whisper, *Joy! Joy! Joy!*

6. February 15, 2006. In the past ten years I've lived in five different states, jumping from newspaper job to newspaper job with the occasional vagabond break to fritter away time in the backcountry. I've had lots of boyfriends. Lots of roommates. A futon mattress that fits in the back of my truck. Last fall I turned thirty, moved to Boulder, declared my roots planted. Most of my friends are married. Many are pregnant. I'm still single.

This morning I'm awake at sunrise, heavy with self-doubt. The night before, I asked a man I really like to leave, even though he cooked me an elaborate Valentine's dinner and clearly wanted to stay. It's complicated. Jeff isn't exactly single, isn't exactly in a relationship. I want a real boyfriend.

As the first light of day illuminates the sky, I lace up my running shoes. My regular loop, 5 miles on a trail that weaves through an open meadow before climbing about one thousand feet to the halfway point, is more punishing than usual. My legs would prefer to shuffle. My lungs have forgotten how to do their job. I press on, hopeful it will get easier. It doesn't. I want to walk, and sometimes I do; being disciplined last night was hard enough.

After climbing for what feels like a year, the trail loops down a canyon and curves into wide switchbacks that cross the broadening valley. With gravity's assist, I relax into the effort. First, it simply feels less painful. Eventually I stop thinking and simply run. I'm rewarded with endorphins that remind me of how my stomach flipped the night before, when Jeff hugged me goodnight. I recall all of the excitement and none of the frustration. It's actually quite simple, I realize. I like Jeff, and he likes me. Things will work out however they are meant to be. To be clear, this is not my natural default. Normally my monkey mind churns and worries and works against me. But this morning my arms pump, and I surge with strength.

By the time I glide home, I've remembered this: Sometimes the simple act of putting one foot in front of the other is all you need to see the world anew.

7. On the day of our wedding, Jeff and I ran one-and-a-half miles up Bear Mountain Trail, a wide path that leads to the base of the Rocky Mountain foothills. It was a sunny summer morning, and the trail forged through a rocky area we'd earlier dubbed "Mountain Lion Lookout." Everyone knows there are wild cats up there, and even if you didn't believe, the severed deer limbs provide ample evidence. We assume mountain lions watch us run, but we've never seen one. They're so elusive.

Jeff and I love this aspect of our life, being so close to the wild, teetering on the verge of control. That's one reason we picked this trail for this special morning. Sure, nothing happens, but that's not the point. The point is something could have happened. Actually, the point is even if something happened, we would have been in it together. Yes, that's definitely the point.

8. I tried to run during my first pregnancy, but stopped early on. I told myself I'd be back once my baby was born and my ligaments and joints didn't wobble and my pubic symphysis, that horrendous shooting pain in my pelvic area, disappeared. Instead of running, I walked. I walked as my stomach grew. I walked up to my due date and two weeks past it. I walked into the hospital in labor and walked the halls. I walked until contractions forced me to stop. I wanted to run away from the hospital, but instead I was eventually rolled into the operating room for an unplanned C-section.

When I got postpartum clearance to exercise, I did the runner's equivalent of going straight for the jugular. I signed up for a trail half-marathon that climbed from eight thousand feet above sea level to ten thousand feet. I had six months to train—piece of cake!–and that training became the scaffolding of my life.

After sleepless nights with a fussy baby, I still rose and laced up my shoes. On weekends I would nurse, drive to the trailhead, knock out a ten-miler, and race home to feed the ravenous beast that had taken over my life. I complained to my friends, most of whom had kids older than mine, about how hard this was. And by *this* I meant everything: motherhood, marriage, exercise. They promised it would get easier. I hated when they said that. I couldn't fathom a day when anything would get easier, when the baby would sleep through the night, the laundry would not stack up, the work would get done, the idea of cooking a meal wouldn't make me want to cry, and the prospect of a run was something I could anticipate, not dread.

Here's how the race went: We were late to the start, which meant I furiously pumped milk while the baby cried in his car seat and Jeff kept both eyes on the road and his foot on the gas pedal. I grabbed my number at registration just as the gun went off. My wave of runners swarmed that steep start. I walked, my head light from the thin air, the stress. By the time the terrain leveled out, I began to jog and secured a spot in the middle of a train of runners. It hurt. I forgot to look at the scenery, to take in the golden aspen leaves, the towering peaks in the distance. Around mile 7, the trail began to gradually climb. By then the urge to quit—not just walk, but to lie down and crawl under a rock and cry until I was all cried out—overwhelmed me, and I gasped out loud. I looked around, hopeful one of my fellow runners would cheer me on. Instead a stick-like waif called out "Trail!" and blazed past.

I made a choice and did what runners do. I put one foot in front of the other and took it mile by incremental mile. I wish I could say it got easier, but it didn't. No matter. I still crossed the finish line, exhausted but triumphant.

Then I realized Jeff and the baby weren't there. He would later feel terrible about their absence, despite his very legitimate excuse of not wanting to wake the napping baby. He would keep apologizing even after I told him it was fine. I didn't mind. I hadn't run the race so my husband and my baby could applaud me at the end. I ran it because I had to. It was the only way I would know who I was, I said. The only way I knew to bridge the life that was with the life I had now.

9. This morning I ran 6 miles under a stunning blue sky. When I got home, I realized it hadn't hurt at all. The miles were smooth and steady, like they were twenty years ago in high school. I didn't think of the kids—or the three interruptions to my sleep last night —or the effort it took to propel myself uphill. I just ran.

I've recalibrated. The trails are the same; the Colorado sky and the bright sun haven't changed. Maybe it's me. Possibly I'm stronger or more impervious to pain. Or, perhaps, running is simply getting easier because I've made a commitment and am sticking to it. Not that I had a choice.

After all, running for me is my truest sport.

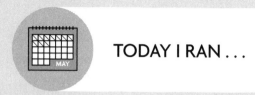

TODAY I RAN . . .

"Because I can."

—ILYSE

"Around the town, on the trails, by the lake, up the hills. I just ran and ran. Kind of like a mother runner version of Forrest Gump—but in a cuter outfit."

—JODI

"Three miles before the sun or my family was awake."

—BECKY

"Six miles; it seemed like a better alternative than watching *Frozen* for the umpteenth time."

—PATRICIA

"My very first half-marathon, under my goal time!"

—ANN

"To do something for myself."

—JAMIE

"Five miles for the first time in my life."

—ALEXIS

"Around like a chicken with its head cut off. Sometimes, that's the only run I can fit in."

—PAURENIA

"Even though I didn't want to."

—KIMBERLY

_____

"In my dreams. Stupid broken foot."

—DEANNA

_____

"A loop I could run blindfolded."

—LEAH

_____

"To soothe my soul and find the peace only running can bring."

—JEN

_____

"Smart. Wanted 10 miles, stopped at 7 because of hip pain."

—SARAH

_____

"Our local community 5K with my husband. Date nights have morphed into date morning races."

—NICOLE

_____

"My longest, hardest run ever."

—LESLIE

_____

"Even though I really didn't feel like it."

—JENNY

_____

"With my seven-year-old twin daughters on scooters beside me."

—KELLY

_____

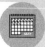

"My first 4 miles without a walk break since baby number three was born twelve weeks ago."

—JULIE

"With heat, humidity, and a teething ten-month-old."

—KRYSTY

"Out of time. Working fourteen-hour days does that, but I will get there. I will."

—JACQUIE

"A 5K in 28:27 at twenty-nine weeks pregnant with baby boy number three."

—KARA

"Three miles on the treadmill; sometimes the last moments of daylight coincide with story time for the kids."

—SARAH

"About ten feet and had to stop due to cramping Achilles tendon."

—JENNY

"A 5K with my six-year-old son: his first!"

—AMANDA

"To cope with dropping my eighteen-year-old daughter off at college."

—TRICIA

"A few blocks around my neighborhood because I only had ten minutes."

—ALICIA

"Ten death-march miles with three bathroom stops. Not fun."

—CATHRYN

"Away from a humongous Great Dane who decided to join me in the street."

—MARCIA

"At 5:00 in the morning so the rest of the day I could be Mom.'"

—AMY

"Four-and-a-half fast, gossip-filled miles with an amazing woman who made me run outside of my comfort zone."

—HEATHER

"My first training run for my comeback 13.1. Kickin' cancer's butt!"

—STACEY

"Nowhere: Last night, I thought I was twenty-one again, drank too much, and stayed out too late."

—MELANIE

"A 5K around Graceland with Elvis impersonators."

—AMY

"Behind, with, then away from my husband in a 10K race!"

—CHARLOTTE

"My seventh half-marathon and a PR!"

—EMELIE

"For my five-year-old son who passed away."

—CARISA

_____

"Because I never want to look back and say, 'I should have run.'"

—ZULMA

_____

"Fifteen miles without even flinching."

—BETHANY

_____

"My hilly route; it makes me feel alive!"

—EMILY

_____

"Nowhere, sadly. This eight-month-old baby bump is just too heavy. . . ."

—PAM

_____

"On an indoor track since it's summer in Arizona."

—JENNIFER

_____

"To get away from the stress of raising a special needs child."

—JULIE

_____

"To silence my own self-doubt."

—EMILY

_____

"Eight miles to get to Dunkin' Donuts."

—JULIE

_____

"Because I need to get back into the swing of it after several months of a pity party."

—CHRISTI

_____

"With my best friend since sixth grade in the pitch dark on a crushed limestone trail."

—BECKY

_____

"Faster than a turtle slogging through peanut butter: success."

—JENNIFER

_____

"My first triathlon . . . holy crap: a triathlon!"

—BRITNEY

_____

"My first sub-11-minute mile. Ever."

—SANDRA

_____

"Because that's what I do every morning. It's a part of my daily routine and who I am."

—TIA

_____

"With two friends, one dog, and a beautiful sunrise during the last mile."

—DIMITY

_____

"And laughed with my best running friend, Molly."

—SBS

_____

TALES FROM ANOTHER MOTHER RUNNER: AUTHOR BIOGRAPHIES

"I have two proudest running accomplishments. One is completing a 50-mile trail ultramarathon. It took freaking forever, but it was pure triumph to cross the line. The second is the first time I ran with all three of my children across the Golden Gate Bridge, a major milestone after years of sweating behind baby joggers. Glorious."

—KRISTIN ARMSTRONG (Author of seven books including *Mile Markers: The 26.2 Most Important Reasons Why Women Run*; contributing editor for *Runner's World*; has written for publications from *Glamour* to *USA Today*; blogs at runnersworld.com/mile-markers-kristin-armstrong.)

"Running has always been about moving through nature, going deep into the wilderness on my own two feet. Whether I'm going out for a solo run in the mountains or journeying across the Grand Canyon, it's an emotional journey as much as a physical one, less like training and more like traveling. Nature is so healing and restorative, give me dirt over asphalt any day."

—KATIE ARNOLD (Creator of Raising Rippers blog on Outside Online; contributor to *Outside*, *Runner's World*, assorted anthologies, and many national publications; at work on a memoir about ultrarunning as a path through grief; blogs at writingfromthenest.blogspot.com.)

"My mantra is 'Just Keep Moving Forward.' Those four little words have carried me through so many tough runs and races—and life events, for that matter. I look at it this way: As long as I am going *forward*, I will get where I need to be. Eventually. Although I have run hills so steep in my neighborhood that the mantra turned into 'Just Don't Fall the Hell Over.' That one works, too."

—MEREDITH ATWOOD (Author of *Triathlon for the Every Woman*; contributor to *Triathlete Magazine*; blogs at SwimBikeMom.com.)

"During a recent half-marathon in Chicago, an unexpected bathroom stop at around mile 7 messed up what I thought had been outstanding pace. Finally, around mile nine-ish, I felt like I was back where I should be pace-wise. I'm a big fan of mantras, and said out loud at least five times: 'Right here. Right here. Right here. Right here.' That phrase—and saying it out loud—really helped me rally and finish the course, despite the potty break, in *under two hours*!"

—AMY BAILEY (Journalist for more than 16 years, with stints at The Associated Press and newspapers in suburban Philadelphia and Green Bay, Wisconsin; blogs at amytherunner.blogspot.com.)

"My grandma once saw me come in from a good run on the country roads near her house and observed, 'I think exercise is the cure for everything.' She was a wise woman, and I miss her all the time."

—TERZAH BECKER (Reporter and editor at the *Wall Street Journal* and *Denver Post* before becoming a librarian.)

"During the winter last year, I noticed an elderly man on my route. He was shuffling along, with an obvious and engrained limp. I saw him several more mornings after that. Impressed, I always nodded ('Just Do It, Sir!') whenever I spotted him. Twice, I even snapped a 'runshot' of him as I closed in on him. I changed routes and my running times, and lost track of my old shuffling man. A couple weekends ago this summer, I spotted him up ahead, carrying a closed umbrella. I was pulling out my phone to snap a, 'hey, my buddy's back,' pic, but decided to go one better: I stopped, introduced myself, told him he's an inspiration, and asked if he would mind if we took a selfie (*usie!*) together. He obliged, and I wrapped my arm around him."

—NICOLE BLADES (Journalist for 18 years and who has written for *Women's Health, Cosmopolitan, MORE, ESPN the Magazine,* and NYTimes.com, among others. Currently working on a new novel; her first novel, *Earth's Waters,* was published in 2007; blogs at MsMaryMack.com.)

"I PR'd in a 5K on the Big Island in Hawaii. I was feeling so good about myself . . . then in the last 100 meters, I was passed by an eight-year-old with an untied shoelace."

—ALISA BONSIGNORE (Writes for healthcare and tech companies; blogs at WhatWouldBettyDo.com.)

"I feel most at home on the trails in northern Michigan, and especially badass when running in tough weather. I'll take a blizzard over a scorcher any day, and running the trails during a downpour is pure bliss."

—HEATHER JOHNSON DUROCHER (A former newspaper reporter for dailies in Michigan, Ohio, and Minnesota; contributor to national magazines including *USA Weekend, Runner's World,* and *Health*; blogs at michiganrunnergirl.com.)

"I was so desperate for a bagel with peanut butter the morning of the Miami Half-Marathon my husband got in the service elevator at the hotel, barged uninvited into the frantic, backed-up, race-day kitchen, and got one for me. My hero."

—JENNY EVERETT (Former Fitness Editor at *Women's Health,* health blogger at *SELF*; writes a food column for *Garden & Gun*; her work has also appeared in, among other places, *Runner's World, O: The Oprah Magazine,* and *Popular Science*; blogs at cookingforsam.com.)

"When my daughter was a year and a half old, she spotted me nearing the finish of a trail marathon before my husband or any of our friends did. Without saying a word to anybody, she grabbed a medal from someone who'd finished before me and ran out onto the course, pointing and yelling 'Mommy!' until she got my attention—and that of nearly every spectator. No race—no Ironman or TransRockies or anything else that I've ever done—has had as sweet a finish as that one."

—MARIT FISCHER (Twenty years' worth of public relations and marketing copywriting; contributed to a couple of magazines that don't exist anymore; has written a children's book "that nobody but my daughter and friends will ever see.")

"Reality is highly overrated when it comes to anything, but especially when it comes to running. There are times I feel like a freakin' gazelle on the road. Don't dare tell me my shadow more closely resembles a walrus. Don't need to know."

—JENNIFER GRAHAM (Op-ed columnist for *The Boston Globe*, and author of *Honey, Do You Need a Ride? Confessions of a Fat Runner*; blogs at jennifergraham.com.)

"I ran my first marathon in New York City in 1989, and have been going long ever since—almost always with friends. My longest race was South Africa's misleadingly named Comrades Marathon, which is actually 56 miles. My knees are fine."

—TISH HAMILTON (Executive editor of *Runner's World*; previous editorial stints at *Rolling Stone, Outside*, and *Sports Illustrated Women*.)

"I once ran a 10K sock-less because I forgot to pack my socks. I ran another one wearing cotton socks because I packed the wrong socks. Neither of these are my proudest moments."

—NICOLE KNEPPER (A licensed clinical professional counselor and author of *Moms Who Drink and Swear: True Tales of Loving My Kids While Losing My Mind*; contributor to numerous humor anthologies, the *Washington Post*, the *Chicago Tribune*, among others; blogs at momswhodrinkandswear.com.)

"I peed in my shorts during my first 5K because my bladder muscles were not up to both the excitement and the downhills."

—ADRIENNE MARTINI (Author of two memoirs: *Hillbilly Gothic* and *Sweater Quest*; blogs at martinimade.com.)

"I've always thought there should be separate age groups for mother runners. For example: age 30-34, 1 to 2 kids; age 30-34, 3 to 4 kids; age 30-34, 5+ kids. I'll start lobbying for those now that we've finished this book."

—DIMITY MCDOWELL (Co-author of *Run Like a Mother + Train Like a Mother* and co-chief mother runner at Another Mother Runner; sports + fitness writer whose work has appeared in *Real Simple, Runner's World*, and others.)

"Four things about my running: 1. I have to chew gum while I run. 2. My husband drilled sheet metal screws into the soles of my running shoes so that I could run outside on ice. 3. I suffered from chronic pain in my lower back during my runs until I began practicing yoga. Bonus: The zen helps when living with all men! 4. I surprised myself twice in 2010 with PRs in races. I have been chasing them unsuccessfully ever since."

—BETHANY MEYER (Contributions in *This Is Childhood, I Just Want to Pee Alone*, and *I Just Want to Be Alone*; columnist at WhatToExpect.com; blogs at bethanymeyer.com, which is also known as I Love Them Most When They're Sleeping.)

"My joy and satisfaction with running rises in direct proportion to my irritation with the laundry pile: The more I run, the more stuff I have to hang dry. It's a vicious cycle. Mountains of dirty workout gear, though, are worth the giddy feeling I get from hearing my kid yell, 'Go, Mama, Go!' as I head out the door to run—or hearing it when I saw her cheering at mile 23 of the New York City Marathon. I mean, there's just nothing better in the world."

—ALISON OVERHOLT (Editor-in-Chief of *espnW*; previous editorial stints at *Seventeen, ESPN The Magazine*, and *Fast Company*; writing has appeared everywhere from *Cosmopolitan* to *O: The Oprah Magazine* to *Fortune*.)

"My favorite gear for long, cold runs is fingerless mittens. When I warm up, I can slip my thumbs out and just push them up my arms."

—SUSAN SCHORN (author of *Smile at Strangers*; writes Bitchslap, a monthly column at McSweeneys.net; also contributes to The Hairpin and the Rumpus, among others.)

"I'm training for my twelfth marathon, and I'm oddly proud I've never run the same 26.2 twice. I'll make an exception for Boston now that I've requalified."

—SARAH BOWEN SHEA (Co-author of *Run Like a Mother + Train Like a Mother* and co-chief mother runner at Another Mother Runner; former freelance writer for publications including *SELF, Real Simple*, and the *New York Times*.)

"I live in Boulder, Colorado, a place with more Olympians-in-training per capita than any place on earth. It's humbling."

—MICHELLE THEALL (Author of the memoir *Teaching the Cat to Sit*, as well as two health and fitness books; editor-in-chief of *Alaska* magazine; blogs at michelletheall.com.)

"I have combined my love for writing and fitness for practical purposes, such as penning a few books, as well as necessities for the running life, such as persuading race directors to let me in an already closed race. In rhyme. Yes, I wrote poetry to get into a race. Not just any race, the epic and notoriously difficult to enter Dipsea Race. It worked."

—KARA DOUGLASS THOM (Author of the Go! Go! Sports Girls series of children's books, as well as the books *See Mom Run; Hot (Sweaty) Mamas: Five Secrets to Life as a Fit Mom;* and *Becoming an Ironman: First Encounters with the Ultimate Endurance Event*. She blogs at lifeasafitmom.com.)

"My favorite routine in life is to wake up at 5:30, and meet my two running partners on the local trails. Sometimes it's too much for me to keep up with my speedy companions, and other times I'm leading the way. Either way, I have to be sick, injured, or in my third trimester to miss this weekly ritual."

—RACHEL WALKER (Has been a daily newspaper reporter, magazine editor, and freelance writer and has written for the *New York Times, Skiing*, babble.com, *Runner's World*, and others; blogs at spawnandsurvive.com.)

ACKNOWLEDGMENTS

It feels odd for two people to write an acknowledgments page when this book was the team effort of hundreds and hundreds; a remarkable number of remarkable women contributed to these pages. Yes, we organized, edited, and assembled the pieces, but scores of you handed us the (honest, funny, poignant, sassy) parts. Without access to your miles, your journeys, your lives, we wouldn't have agonized for days over the best words to write on this page. (A good place to be in, we realize . . . still surprisingly tough.)

So a huge thanks for sharing your stories about tempo runs and temper tantrums, first steps and finish lines—and, in doing so, cementing the amazing community that is Another Mother Runner. We are so grateful.

Thanks to the twenty talented writers who contributed their stories—and put up with what sometimes must have felt like endless editing requests. Bethany Meyer, Heather Johnson Durocher, Adrienne Martini, and Jennifer Graham took on other to-do tasks; we appreciate you going above and beyond. Katie Oglesby (aka the ultrarunner who didn't meet the 30-hour race cutoff) was also instrumental in helping us pull off this tome. The support from Kristin Barnett, Denise Dollar, and Jonna Bass Parr was integral as we stepped on the gas for the final mile. As always, we want to give credit to the smart, talented book women who find our words a home and bring them to life: Jane Dystel, Chris Schillig, and Kathy Hilliard.

Our families—Grant, Amelia, and Ben for Dimity; Jack, Phoebe, John, and Daphne for SBS—nicely put up with us through months of book assembly. (Except for that one time when Ben walked into Dimity's office and asked, "Who is the boss of this mother runner thing anyway?" She said she was. "Then why do you work so hard?")

Last but not least, Dimity's posse of neighborhood BRFs and Sarah's BRF, Molly, kept us accountable and laughing through countless miles. Which, of course, just means we'll always have plenty more stories to tell.

XO—Dimity + Sarah

Notes • Things to Remember

Notes + Things to Remember

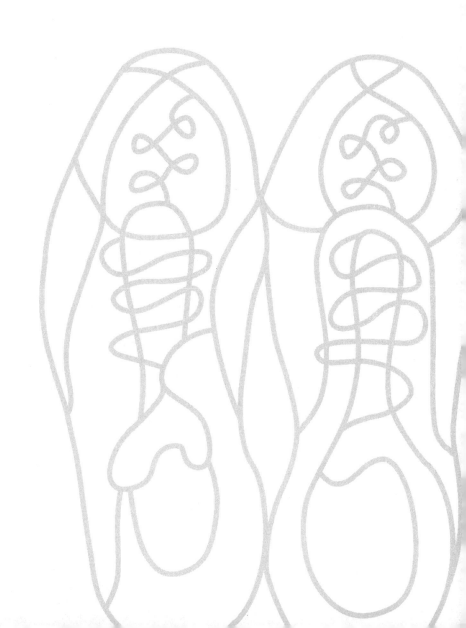

Notes + Things to Remember

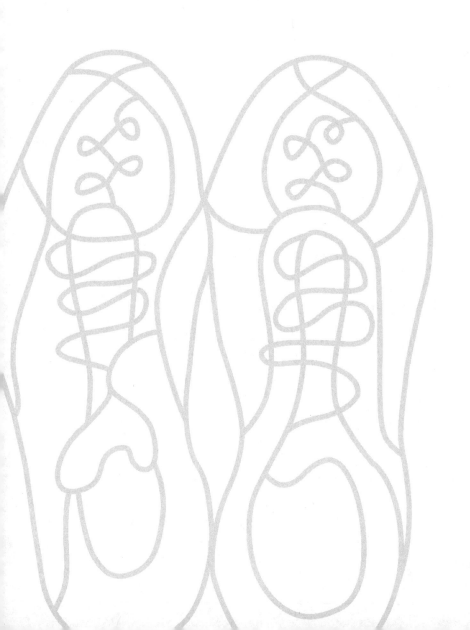

Notes + Things to Remember

Andrews McMeel Publishing, LLC
an Andrews McMeel Universal company
1130 Walnut Street, Kansas City, Missouri 64106

www.andrewsmcmeel.com

15 16 17 18 19 RR4 10 9 8 7 6 5 4 3 2 1

ISBN: 978-1-4494-4990-2

Library of Congress Control Number: 2014949996

Editor: Chris Schillig
Art director and designer: Julie Barnes
Production editor: Maureen Sullivan
Production manager: Cliff Koehler
Demand planner: Sue Eikos

Lyrics from "Son's Gonna Rise" by Citizen Cope. Copyright © 2004 by Arista Records. Reprinted by permission.

Lyrics from "I Will Wait" by Mumford & Sons. Copyright © 2012 by Universal Island Records, a division of Universal Music Operations Limited. Reprinted by permission.

ATTENTION: SCHOOLS AND BUSINESSES
Andrews McMeel books are available at quantity discounts with bulk purchase for educational, business, or sales promotional use. For information, please e-mail the Andrews McMeel Publishing Special Sales Department: specialsales@amuniversal.com.